# schiZophRENiA

# schiZophRENiA

## seven approaches

Arnold H. Buss and
Edith H. Buss, editors

Routledge
Taylor & Francis Group
LONDON AND NEW YORK

First published 1969 by Transaction Publishers

2 Park Square, Milton Park, Abingdon, Oxfordshire OX14 4RN
711 Third Avenue, New York, NY 10017

*Routledge is an imprint of the Taylor & Francis Group, an informa business*

First issued in hardback 2017



Library of Congress Catalog Number: 2008002633

Library of Congress Cataloging-in-Publication Data

Theories of schizophrenia.
Schizophrenia : seven approaches / [edited by] Arnold H. Buss and Edith H. Buss.
p. ; cm.
Originally published: Theories of schizophrenia. 1st ed. New York : Atherton Press, 1969.
Includes bibliographical references and indexes.
ISBN 978-0-202-36230-4 (alk. paper)
1. Schizophrenia. I. Buss, Arnold H., 1924- II. Buss, Edith H. III. Title.
[DNLM: 1. Schizophrenia. 2. Psychological Theory. WM 203 T396s 1969a]

RC514.B87 2008
616.89'8—dc22 2008002633

ISBN 13: 978-0-202-36230-4 (pbk)
ISBN 13: 978-1-138-53223-6 (hbk)

# *Contents*

# *Introduction*

ARNOLD H. BUSS
EDITH H. BUSS

Schizophrenia is one of the most common and most severe kinds of psychopathology. For more than a hundred years investigators have struggled with the problem, attempting to understand the nature and origins of a set of symptoms that occurs in roughly one person in a hundred. As there are many points of view about psychopathology, so there are many theories of schizophrenia. This book includes seven theories of schizophrenia, a sampling of biological, psychological, and sociological approaches.

This chapter introduces these theories by briefly answering the following questions. What is the nature of schizophrenia? What models of man are implicitly assumed by the theories? What general approach does each theory represent? What does each theory assume, what evidence does it require for proof, and what follows if the theory is correct?

## The Nature of Schizophrenia

Most clinicians agree that schizophrenia includes two kinds of symptoms: those concerning *cognition* and those concerning *social withdrawal*. The cognitive symptoms are:

1. disturbances of language and thought
2. distortions of the body image
3. a retreat from reality to fantasy
4. hallucinations
5. delusions.

The symptoms of social withdrawal are:

1. fear of others
2. avoidance of relationships with others
3. isolation from others.

These two classes of symptoms may cause trouble for any theory attempting to explain schizophrenia: a given theory may explain one set of symptoms but be hard pressed to account for the other. Consider a theory that establishes the family as the basic cause of schizophrenia. A child might be treated so badly and so inconsistently that he eventually becomes schizophrenic, presumably having learned to fear others, to avoid them, and finally to shut himself off from them. The theory would neatly account for the symptoms of social withdrawal but not for the cognitive symptoms; that would require assumptions beyond those needed to explain the symptoms of social withdrawal.

This problem is not restricted to theories that focus on the family as a cause of schizophrenia. It is a source of difficulty for any theory of schizophrenia. Because schizophrenia includes diverse symptoms, any theory must account for a range of behavior, not merely one or a few. Stated in broader terms, the issue concerns the nature of schizophrenia. Is it a single ailment like arthritis? Or is it a combination of equally mysterious ailments like cancer? Probably the latter.

Schizophrenia does not stand alone as a psychosis easily distinguished from other psychoses. Rather, it may be considered as the end point of three different dimensions of psychosis (see Figure 1). In this context, there is a basic, nuclear schizophrenia which corresponds to what Kraepelin labeled *dementia praecox*, or, in modern terminology, *true schizophrenia*: classical symptoms of thought disorder and autism with a poor prognosis. Related to this central psychosis are three other psychoses the mixed forms of which have schizophrenic-like symptoms.

*1. Depression.* At one end of this dimension (see Figure 1) is psychotic depression, the major feature of which is of course melancholia. At the other end is nuclear schizophrenia, which is marked by the absence of affect—also called *flattened affect.* There are also mixed forms occupying the middle of the dimension. These manifest a combination of thought disorder *and* depressive affect; hence the term *schizoaffective.*

2. *Atypical Psychosis.* At one end of this dimension is a group of psychoses that includes cyclic psychoses (Leonhard, 1961), nonprocess psychoses (Stephens and Astrup, 1963), and pseudoneurotic schizophrenia (Hoch and Polatin, 1949). They are called atypical because they differ from nuclear schizophrenia (the basic or *typical* psychosis) as follows: onset is sudden and symptoms are acute, there is much confusion and disorientation, little intellectual deficit, and prognosis is good. Onset in nuclear schizophrenia, in contrast, is typically slow, symptoms are chronic, there is no confusion or disorientation, much intellectual deficit, and prognosis is poor. There are also mixed forms occupying the middle of the dimension, having features of both nuclear schizophrenia and the atypical psychoses.

*3. Paranoia.* At one end of this dimension is paranoia. Strictly speaking, paranoia is not a psychosis, but a nonpsychotic *monomania*. The paranoiac has a fixed delusional sys-

**Figure 1**

**Schizophrenia in Relation to Other Psychoses**

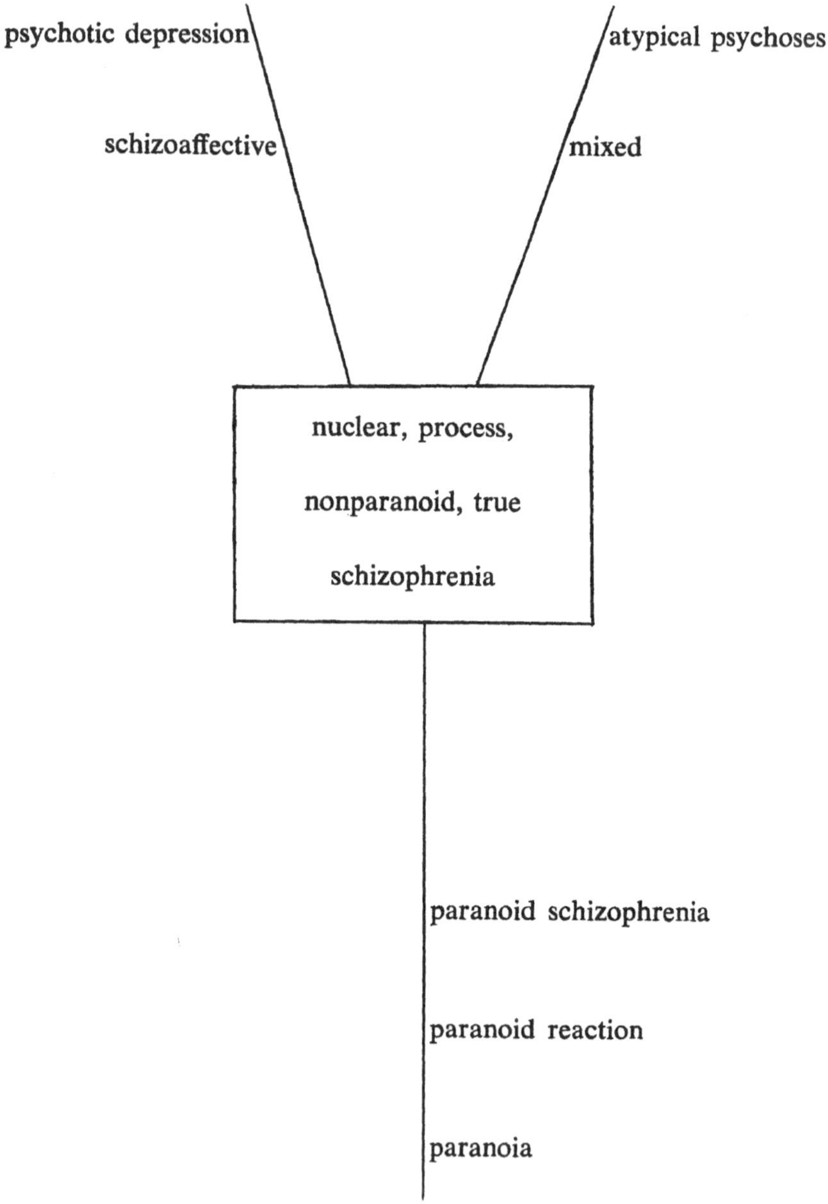

tem based on a faulty premise. The delusional system is usually sufficiently encapsulated so that it does not intrude greatly into everyday interactions with others. Moving in from this extreme, we come to *paranoid reaction,* a psychosis marked by extreme suspiciousness, little thought disorder, and slightly systematized delusions. It is but a short step to *paranoid schizophrenia,* which is characterized by suspiciousness, some thought disorder, and unsystematized delusions (grandiose or hostile). From this point, we move to the end of the dimension—nuclear, nonparanoid schizophrenia, which is marked by thought disorder, psychological deficit, poor prognosis, but no delusions.

Thus three dimensions of psychosis are conceptualized with nuclear schizophrenia at the core and the dimensions radiating outward. There are mixed forms, intermediate between nuclear schizophrenia and the ends of the three dimensions. Some of these combinations have enough of the features of nuclear schizophrenia to be included under the heading of schizophrenia—paranoid schizophrenia and schizoaffective psychosis, for example. They are troublesome for any theory of schizophrenia. If the theory is genetic, does the same inherited defect lead to both paranoid schizophrenia and schizoaffective psychosis? If the theory is social, does the same family environment lead to both paranoid and nonparanoid schizophrenia? Any theory that attempts to answer these questions must add assumptions, thereby becoming complex and perhaps cumbersome.

## Models of Man

All theories of schizophrenia implicitly assume a particular model of man. They all make an underlying assumption about the nature of man—specifically, that aspect of his life deemed to be crucial. Accordingly, there are three models of man, each focusing on that aspect the theory emphasizes in attempting to explain schizophrenia: biological, psychological, or social.

### *Biological Man*

Man may be viewed as a biochemical system interacting with the environment. His fundamental task is to extract from the environment the physical and chemical requirements of life: oxygen, food, water, and so on. Beyond this, he must take in and process large amounts of information, an activity that requires that his senses and nervous system function well. The nervous system underlies all behavior and must therefore be anatomically and physiologically intact to insure normal, adjustive behavior.

Anatomical defects in the nervous system may be gross (a malformed spinal cord for instance) or minute (such as certain types of improperly constructed neurons). Physiological dysfunction occurs when the substances underlying neural transmission (*neurohumors*) are insufficient, persist too long, or are metabolized incorrectly and form substances that interfere with neural functioning. Another possibility is a chemical imbalance among the various neurohumors, which might upset the delicate feedback mechanisms operating among the various functioning parts of the nervous system.

The nervous system, in both anatomical and physiological aspects, is inherited along with all the other parts of our bodies. We can inherit a normal, adequately functioning nervous system, which leads to essentially normal behavior; or we can inherit a nervous system which, no matter how slight the flaw, does not function as it should and therefore leads to deviant behavior, e.g., schizophrenia.

### *Psychological Man*

Man may be viewed as a *behaving* organism, responding to environmental stimuli with sequences of acts. He needs to take in information and process it, focusing on essentials and avoiding minor distractions. He must be able to sort out important from nonessential stimuli, attending to the former and screening out the latter. He must also be capable of altering this selective attention when the situation demands it. In brief, man must have normal *cognitive* functioning: the proper perception, processing, and encoding of information.

Another aspect of psychological man concerns *motivation,* specifically anxiety. Our world is a potentially destructive place, if not of our tissues, then of our self-esteem. We must contend with the dangers of bodily harm, rejection by those we care for, loss in competition, and loss of status. The developing child learns what to fear, the signals that warn of danger, and of the need to escape from or cope with the oncoming danger.

In the face of these various threats, man's task is to hold down his level of anxiety. He must maintain at least some equanimity in the face of danger or unpleasantness. If he can keep himself from going to pieces, he should be able to make responses that reduce the danger or avoid the negative consequences. The alternative is to panic and sleepwalk through a living nightmare, giving up the struggle and avoiding all possible sources of anxiety, especially other persons, by isolating oneself. The extreme of panic, surrender, and isolation is represented by schizophrenia.

We have been viewing man's behavior at any given time, but all behavior occurs in the context of the individual's life cycle. Each of us walks the path from infancy to maturity, passing through sequential phases or eras. Thus, man may be considered a growing organism, with growth defined in psychological, not biological, terms. Normal development consists of moving through sequential stages during the periods of infancy, childhood, and adolescence to arrive at the endpoint of maturity in adulthood. As development proceeds, the individual must give up earlier, outmoded responses for newer, appropriate responses. For example, in relating to others he must progress from a predominantly childlike role of depend-ence to a predominantly peer role of equality. This process of surrendering less mature for more mature behavior occurs repeatedly during the developmental sequence. The normal adult has discarded his earlier childlike behavior and there is little of it in his repertoire; the immature adult still has large residuals of childhood in his behavioral repertoire. The deviant adult has progressed some of the way toward maturity but has gone back to behaviors typical of earlier stages. This is called *regression*, which, when it occurs to an extreme degree, results in schizophrenia.

## *Social Man*

Man is obviously a social organism. As an infant, he cannot survive without the tender care of a mother. Thereafter he is tutored in the ways of his group and society. This socialization occurs mainly in the family and is conducted by mother, father, siblings, and relatives. Beyond the family are larger social groups and classes, and ultimately there is society as a whole. Each individual matures and moves out of his immediate family group into the wider spaces of society. Each segment or class of society differs in degree of organization and in the rewards held out to individual members; and both the segments and the totality are changeable, shifting slowly as time passes.

If society is reasonably stable and offers sufficient rewards to its members, and if the family completes its job of socialization without excessive anxiety or alienation, the outcome should be a normal, mature, socialized adult. If society is disorganized or nonrewarding, or if the family is inconsistent and rejecting during the process of socialization, the outcome should be an abnormal, immature, partly-socialized adult. Presumably, if family or society, or both, are sufficiently vicious, the ultimate outcome should be schizophrenia.

## Theories of Schizophrenia

We shall discuss seven theories of schizophrenia. Each one implicitly assumes a model of man: biological, psychological, or social. There is one biological theory: it focuses on genetic and neurological aspects. There are four psychological theories: one focuses on cognitive functioning, one on motivation, and two on regression. And there are two social theories: one focuses on the family and the other on social forces beyond the family.

### *Genetic-Neural*

The biological approach to schizophrenia has generated two kinds of theories. The first is the *genetic theory,* which assumes that schizophrenia is an inherited biological disposition. The second is the *neural theory,* which assumes that the cause of schizophrenia is malfunction of the nervous system. The two kinds of theory have been combined into a single theory by Meehl (1962). We have included his formulation (Chapter 1) because it is the most complete biological approach, encompassing both genetic and neural aspects.

Meehl's assumptions are straightforward. First, there is an inherited defect that predisposes the individual to schizophrenia. Second, this defect resides in the nervous system, specifically in the functioning of individual neurons. Third, schizophrenia is a disease similar to other biological diseases. As an example to clarify this assumption, consider hay fever. The necessary condition is an inherited biological predisposition that consists of a tendency to overreact to certain kinds of proteins. The sufficient condition consists of certain substances in the environment—specifically pollens or seeds blowing through the air. If an individual with this inherited disposition resides in an area with no pollen or seeds (say, Antarctica), he will not develop hay fever; the sufficient condition is absent. If he resides in a locale that has pollen, he will develop hay fever; both the necessary and sufficient conditions are present. Meehl's theory of schizophrenia makes analogous assumptions: the necessary condition is an inherited defect of the nervous system, and the sufficient condition is an unfortunate early psychological environment. It follows that the more severe the inherited defect, the milder need be the environmental stress to trigger the schizophrenia.

Concerning the inheritance of schizophrenia, there are several theories that specify the precise genetic mechanism. Kallmann (1953) proposes a recessive gene, Böök (1953) suggests a dominant gene, and Weinberg and Lobstein (1943) assume that there is a different gene for each subtype of schizophrenia. None of these theories has been proven (Buss, 1966). Geneticists lean toward the notion of a single gene (dominant or recessive) for schizophrenia, but there is simply not enough evidence to confirm this. The available evidence strongly indicates an inherited component in schizophrenia, but the precise mechanism of inheritance is still in doubt, and Meehl wisely refrains from specifying one.

There are also several theories concerning the neural defect in schizophrenia. An obvious place to search is in the substances that underlie neural transmission, the neurohumors. Woolley (1962) proposed serotonin, a brain neurohumor, as the focal chemical; too much or too little serotonin presumably leads to schizophrenia. Hoffer and Osmond (1959) focus on the metabolic products of adrenaline, a well known neurohumor; an inherited enzyme defect presumably leads to faulty oxydation of adrenaline and the resulting chemicals interfere with brain function, thereby causing symptoms of schizophrenia. Rubin (1962) suggests that schizophrenia is caused by any of several kinds of imbalance between sympathetic nervous functioning (mediated by the neurohumor, adrenaline) and parasympathetic nervous functioning (mediated by the neurohumor, acetylcholine).

Meehl's neural speculations are more closely tied to research in neuropsychology. He locates the neural defect in individual neurons, specifically in the *synapses* between neurons, and it is this that makes Meehl's proposals so interesting: while other neural theories are based mainly on the pharmacological properties of neurohumors, his is based on relationships between behavior and the nervous system. Common to both pharmacological and neuropsychological theories is the assumption that schizophrenia is caused by *faulty biological processes*. The specific learning that occurs during the individual's life—that is, the *content* of the psychosis (the particular hallucination or delusion)—is presumably unimportant. This contrasts sharply with an environmental theory such as the family approach, as we shall see below.

Meehl's theory requires two kinds of evidence to sustain it. First, the precise genetic mechanism of schizophrenia needs to be established. Although Meehl side steps this issue, he does state that the defect is inherited. It is extremely difficult, however, to separate inherited from environmental effects when the same parent who presumably passes on the gene also rears the child. Ultimately the best evidence for any theory involving inheritance is a demonstration of the precise manner in which the trait is passed on from one generation to the next.

Second, the precise nature of the neural defect needs to be established. It may be in the neurohumors, as some investigators have suggested; in individual neurons, as Meehl suggests; or in a combination of these two. But certainly we need to pin down the neural defect if the theory is to be proven.

If Meehl's theory proves to be correct, what follows? One consequence is that the only real means of prevention is through eugenics. Individuals with the taint of schizophrenia would have to be prevented from breeding children, else schizophrenia could never be eliminated. Concerning therapy for schizophrenics, Meehl's theory suggests two possibilities. One is to attempt chemical therapy in an effort to restore normal neural functioning; the other is to try rehabilitation, as would be done with any other neurological condition.

### *Cognitive*

The cognitive approach to schizophrenia emphasizes man as an information processor. The information may come from the senses: we are all familiar with the senses attuned to the environment around us—eyes, ears, skin, nose, and tongue—and less familiar with the senses attuned to the internal environment—the stretch receptors in joints and muscles, for example, that comprise kinesthesis, the sense of movement.

The information may also consist of associations, thoughts, ideas, or memories. Each individual "maps" his psychological world—marking off boundaries among stimuli, establishing similarities among stimuli, and moving conceptually from immediate sense impressions to less concrete ideas and concepts.

A cognitive theorist may lean toward one or another of these aspects of cognition in attempting to explain schizophrenia. He may focus on associations, for it has been clearly demonstrated that schizophrenics have associative disturbances; or he may focus on concepts, for it has been clearly demonstrated that schizophrenics have conceptual disturbances. But underlying these two kinds of cognitive dysfunction is a more fundamental defect in attention—the ability to maintain a set and keep out distracting stimuli. In recent years investigators who view schizophrenia in terms of cognitive dysfunction have increasingly endorsed the notion that attention is the key to understanding schizophrenia.

Shakow (1963) has been active in this area for several decades. He emphasizes maintaining a preparatory set for oncoming stimuli, and he adduces much laboratory evidence to back up this notion. A somewhat broader theory has been formulated by McGhie and Chapman (1961; Chapter 2, this volume), who attempt to integrate not only laboratory evidence but also clinical observations, developmental processes, and the notion of consciousness.

McGhie and Chapman assume that the basic problem in schizophrenia is an inability to select, focus on, and regulate incoming information. Because the schizophrenic simply cannot cope with all the distracting elements in his environment, he becomes perplexed, confused, and inefficient. This primary cognitive deficit thus causes motivational and social problems, for, as his cognitive apparatus fails, the schizophrenic's world changes rapidly. He is puzzled and frightened by his distorted perceptions, and, as his anxiety mounts, he avoids all sources of confused perceptions, especially other persons. He attempts to struggle with his problem alone, or at least to avoid the threatening presence of others. Thus the social-motivational aspects of schizophrenia are viewed as deriving from the more fundamental cognitive aspects.

The evidence for an attentional deficit in schizophrenia is very strong (see Lang and Buss, 1965), but the specific theory of McGhie and Chapman has not been proven. Their theory requires a longitudinal study. Schizophrenics would have to be followed from the earliest symptoms through the period of chronicity, for only then could it be established whether the cognitive dysfunction appears first and then causes a secondary reaction of fear and social withdrawal. To their credit, McGhie and Chapman suggest such a study.

If the theory proves to be true, it will have no bearing on prevention; although there are hints of neural involvement, it does not specify a particular etiology. The theory implies that rehabilitation is all that should be attempted in therapy; the trick would be to simplify the schizophrenic's environment and help him to attend to the salient stimuli. Anything that helps the schizophrenic to shut out distracting stimuli would presumably render him more comfortable and more efficient.

## *Motivation (Anxiety)*

Many clinicians believe that a basic cause of schizophrenia is excessive anxiety. One possibility is that the potential schizophrenic is abnormally sensitive to criticism and rebuff. This is the social censure hypothesis (Garmezy and Rodnick, 1959), which assumes that the schizophrenic's heightened fear of rejection causes him to be inefficient and drives him into a self-imposed isolation from others.

Another possibility is that the potential schizophrenic's high anxiety serves as an irrelevant and interfering *drive.* Mednick (1958; Chapter 3, this volume) has made this assumption in attempting to account for the thinking disorder in schizophrenia. He first assumes that the schizophrenic is extremely anxious and then that high anxiety (high drive) leads to overgeneralization. More and more stimuli come to be frightening, and the person is driven to avoid these stimuli. One way of escaping is to think of remote, irrelevant thoughts and associations. These remote associations distract the schizophrenic from anxiety-provoking thoughts, and his anxiety level is thereby reduced. This reduction in anxiety is rewarding, and the tendency to think irrelevant and distant thoughts becomes habitual.

The evidence bearing on Mednick's theory is conflicting, with both positive and negative findings being reported (see Buss and Lang, 1965). What would settle the issue perhaps is a longitudinal study whereby schizophrenics are followed from the earliest sign of the psychosis until its chronic stages; it might then be seen whether they actually do start out being panicky and then overgeneralize and begin to think irrelevant thoughts, finally dropping in anxiety level as the irrelevant thoughts distract them.

Mednick's theory has little to say about prevention or cure. Prevention would ostensibly focus on minimizing anxiety, but this would hold as well for a wide variety of nonschizophrenics, many of whom are anxious. In attempting a cure, the schizophrenic would presumably be taught not to overgeneralize, but precisely how this might be accomplished is not stated.

### *Regression*

Both psychoanalytic theory and the comparative-developmental approach assume that there are fixed stages in the developmental sequence. Every child must master the problems of a given stage and then proceed to the next one. The end point of the sequence is maturity and normality. Some adults return to behavioral modes characteristic of earlier stages; this is called *regression.* Regression causes immaturity and abnormality, and the severest regression causes the severest abnormality, schizophrenia.

We shall discuss two theories. One derives from the neopsychoanalytic views of Harry Stack Sullivan and the other, from the comparative-developmental approach of Heinz Werner.

*1. Regression: Neopsychoanalytic.* Kantor and Winder (1959; Chapter 4, this volume) have elaborated Sullivan's theory, relating his five stages of early childhood to the process-reactive dimension of schizophrenia. As we noted earlier, process, or nuclear schizophrenia, is the core schizophrenic psychosis; it has a poor prognosis and considerable psychological deficit. Reactive or atypical schizophrenia includes various nonschizophrenic characteristics, and it has a better prognosis and less psychological deficit. Kantor and Winder assume that within schizophrenia there are variations in the depth of regression: the severer the regression, the more *process* is the schizophrenia; the milder the regression, the more *reactive* is the schizophrenia. The details are worked out in terms of Sullivan's five stages.

Kantor and Winder mention some correlational evidence supporting their theory, but the crucial evidence will have to come from a longitudinal study. They focus on infancy and early childhood as the critical phases, and therefore individuals would have to be followed from infancy onward.

If the theory were true, there would be implications for

prevention. The authors are a little vague, but they do imply that the infant must be nurtured and loved, for disapproval and rejection are likely to lead to fixation and subsequently to a schizophrenic regression. There are no suggestions for therapy, although it might be guessed that traditional relationship psychotherapy would be the treatment of choice.

2. *Regression: Comparative-Developmental.* Goldman (1962; Chapter 5, this volume) has applied Heinz Werner's approach (1948) to schizophrenia. The fundamental assumption of the comparative-developmental approach is that development moves from an unorganized, undifferentiated, diffuse state to an organized, differentiated, specific state. The key process in development is differentiation: the proliferation of different response modes and then the organization of these into a hierarchy of behavioral tendencies.

Goldman assumed that schizophrenia represents a regression back to the earliest developmental stages—those characterized by diffusiveness, generalized responsivity, and a lack of differentiation. He set himself the task of demonstrating parallels between children's and schizophrenics' behavior tendencies: presumably, if schizophrenics have regressed, their behavior should resemble that of children. How close the parallels are is debatable (see Buss, 1966, p. 259).

Goldman's theory, like that of Kantor and Winder, offers little in the way of prevention or therapy. His theory is more descriptive than etiological.

### *Family*

Many clinicians have identified the family as the source of schizophrenia. Some believe that the *communication* process underlies the development of schizophrenia. Others believe that *emotional conflicts* within the family can be so traumatic that the patient is driven to schizophrenia. Still others combine the two, believing that schizophrenia is learned in the context of a family with both poor communication and much conflict:

> The schizophrenic patient is more prone to withdraw through his symbolization of reality than other patients, because his foundation in reality is precarious, having been raised amidst irrationality and chronically exposed to intra-familial communications that distort and deny what should be the obvious interpretation of the environment, including the recognition and understanding of impulses and the affective behavior of members of the family (Lidz, *et al.*, 1958, p. 307).

One of the outstanding theories of the family as the cause of schizophrenia is the *double bind* hypothesis of Bateson *et al.* (1956; Chapter 6, this volume). The notion of double bind means that the victim has no responses available that allow him to succeed; he must lose. Concerning the development of schizophrenia, the basic assumption is that the mother places her child in a double bind. The child is tied to the mother by a need for nurturance and love. The mother simulates affection but rejects the child whenever she is approached. The child is confronted with the opposed messages of love and hostility, or approach and avoidance—both emanating from the mother. The situation is worsened by the mother's complete denial of either hostility or opposed messages, and with this she provides a model of irrationality for the child to imitate. The child takes refuge in denial, fantasy, and irrationality, thereby starting down the road to schizophrenia.

The evidence bearing on this theory consists of clinical observations, which appear to support the theory. Unfortunately, control groups are lacking, and it is not entirely clear whether the double bind situation is unique to families of schizophrenics. Furthermore, it is difficult to disentangle the contributions of heredity and environment: the mother who places her child in a double bind may also pass on a hereditary predisposition toward schizophrenia. We shall not easily solve this problem of separating the effects of a vicious family environment from the effects of heredity.

If the theory were true, it would pave the way for the prevention of schizophrenia. The major problem would be to detect mothers (or perhaps even fathers) who involve their children in a double bind situation. The child could then be removed to a foster home and, once outside the original home, would never learn the patterns of irrationality that lead to schizophrenia. The theory says less about cure, although it might recommend a relationship psychotherapy, especially with a benign, maternal therapist.

## *Social Isolation*

A prominent symptom of schizophrenia is social withdrawal, the patient being shy, seclusive, and solitary. How does this condition develop? One possibility is that the child is pushed aside and isolated by the very community in which he resides. This is the basic assumption of Faris' theory (1934; Chapter 7, this volume), which is still influential more than three decades after it was formulated.

Faris argued that being rejected or ignored by fellow members of the community invariably leads to a "shut-in" personality. The individual slowly turns away from social contacts and no longer checks his notions of reality against a social consensus. As his social distance from others increases, he orients his attention more and more toward himself, especially his fantasies and his body. He fails to develop normal social roles or adequate communication skills. He remains outside the mainstream of everyday life and gradually drifts into schizophrenia.

The evidence bearing on the theory is controversial. Faris himself (Faris and Dunham, 1939) collected data relating social disorganization to schizophrenia. But critics (Kennedy, 1964, for example) have pointed out that these and other positive findings are not relevant to the social isolation hypothesis and that there are also negative findings. As with several theories mentioned earlier, the crucial evidence will have to come from a longitudinal study that traces the development of schizophrenia from childhood to the onset of psychotic symptoms.

If the theory were proven true, it would offer a means of preventing schizophrenia. The most fundamental preventive would be to alter social organization, particularly at the community level, in such a way as to prevent individuals from being rejected or ignored by their neighbors. Beyond this, the theory implies that where there is social disorganization, there should be great vigilance in detecting potential isolates. If such individuals could be brought back into the mainstream of community life, presumably they would never become "shut-in" personalities and, subsequently, schizophrenics. As the treatment of choice, Faris suggested relationship therapy. The schizophrenic should be helped to re-establish social contacts, to break out of his isolation, and to take his place in the community—goals probably best accomplished by interpersonal therapy, both individual and group.

## REFERENCES

Bateson, G., D. D. Jackson, J. Haley, and J. Weakland, "Toward a Theory of Schizophrenia," *Behavioral Science,* 1 (1956), 251–64.

Böök, J. A., "Schizophrenia as a Gene Mutation," *Acta Genetica,* 4 (1953), 133–39.

Buss, A. H., *Psychopathology* (New York: John Wiley, 1966).

Buss, A. H. and P. J. Lang, "Psychological Deficit in Schizophrenia. I: Affect, Reinforcement, and Concept Attainment," *Journal of Abnormal Psychology,* 70 (1965), 2–24.

Faris, R. E. L., "Cultural Isolation and the Schizophrenic Personality," *American Journal of Sociology,* 40 (1934), 155–64.

Faris, R. E. L., and H. W. Dunham, *Mental Disorders in Urban Areas* (Chicago: University of Chicago Press, 1939).

Garmezy, N., and E. H. Rodnick, "Premorbid Adjustment and Performance in Schizophrenia: Implications for Interpreting Heterogeneity in Schizophrenia," *Journal of Nervous and Mental Disease,* 129 (1959), 450–66.

Goldman, A. E., "A Comparative-developmental Approach to Schizophrenia," *Psychological Bulletin,* 59 (1962), 57–69.

Hoch, P., and P. Polatin, "Pseudoneurotic Forms of Schizophrenia," *Psychiatric Quarterly,* 23 (1949), 248–76.

Hoffer, A., and H. Osmond, "The Adrenochrome Model and Schizophrenics," *Journal of Nervous and Mental Disease,* 128 (1959), 18–35.

Kallmann, F. J., *Heredity in Health and Mental Disorder* (New York: W. W. Norton, 1953).

Kantor, R. E., and C. Winder, "The Process-reactive Continuum: A Theoretical Proposal," *Journal of Nervous and Mental Disease,* 129 (1959), 429–34.

Kennedy, M. C., "Is There an Ecology of Mental Illness?" *International Journal of Social Psychiatry,* 10 (1964), 119–33.

Lang, P. J., and A. H. Buss, "Psychological Deficit in Schizophrenia: II. Interference and Activation," *Journal of Abnormal Psychology,* 70 (1965), 77–106.

Leonhard, K., "Cycloid Psychoses—Endogenous Psychoses Which Are Neither Schizophrenic Nor Manic-depressive," *Journal of Mental Science,* 107 (1961), 633–48.

Lidz, T., A. R. Cornelison, D. Terry, and S. Fleck, "The Intrafamilial Environment of the Schizophrenic Patient. VI. The Transmission of Irrationality," *Archives of Neurology and Psychiatry,* 79 (1958), 305–16.

McGhie, A., and J. Chapman, "Disorders of Attention and Perception in Early Schizophrenia," *British Journal of Medical Psychology,* 34 (1961), 103–17.

Mednick, S. "A Learning Theory Approach to Research in Schizophrenia," *Psychological Bulletin,* 55 (1958), 316–27.

Meehl, P. E., "Schizotaxia, Schizotypy, Schizophrenia," *American Psychologist,* 17 (1962), 827–38.

Rubin, L. S., "Patterns of Adrenergic-cholinergic Imbalance in the Functional Psychoses," *Psychological Review,* 69 (1962), 501–19.

Shakow, D., "Psychological Deficit in Schizophrenia," *Behavioral Science,* 8 (1963), 275–305.

Stephens, J. H., and C. Astrup, "Prognosis in 'Process' and 'Non-process' Schizophrenia," *American Journal of Psychiatry,* 119 (1963), 945–53.

Weinberg, I., and J. Lobstein, "Inheritance in Schizophrenia," *Acta Psychiatrica Neurologica,* 18 (1943), 93–140.

Werner, H., *Comparative Psychology of Mental Development* (Chicago: Follett, 1948).

Woolley, D. W., *The Biochemical Bases of Psychoses* (New York: John Wiley, 1962).

# 1: *Schizotaxia, Schizotypy, Schizophrenia*

PAUL E. MEEHL

In the course of the last decade, while spending several thousand hours in the practice of intensive psychotherapy, I have treated—sometimes unknowingly except in retrospect—a considerable number of schizoid and schizophrenic patients. Like all clinicians, I have formed some theoretical opinions as a result of these experiences. While I have not until recently begun any systematic research efforts on this baffling disorder, I felt that to share with you some of my thoughts, based though they are upon clinical impressions in the context of selected research by others, might be an acceptable use of this occasion.

Let me begin by asking a question which I find is almost never answered correctly by our clinical students on Ph.D. orals, and the answer to which they seem to dislike when it is offered. Suppose that you were required to write down a procedure for selecting an individual from the population who would be diagnosed as schizophrenic by a psychiatric staff;

Address of the President to the seventieth Annual Convention of the American Psychological Association, St. Louis, September 2, 1962. Reprinted by permission of the author and publisher from *American Psychologist*, 17 (1962), 827–38.

you have to wager $1,000 on being right; you may not include in your selection procedure any behavioral fact, such as a symptom or trait, manifested by the individual. What would you write down? So far as I have been able to ascertain, there is only one thing you could write down that would give you a better than even chance of winning such a bet—namely, "Find an individual X who has a schizophrenic identical twin." Admittedly, there are many other facts which would raise your odds somewhat above the low base rate of schizophrenia. You might, for example, identify X by first finding mothers who have certain unhealthy child-rearing attitudes; you might enter a subpopulation defined jointly in such demographic variables as age, size of community, religion, ethnic background, or social class. But these would leave you with a pretty unfair wager, as would the rule: "Find an X who has a fraternal twin, of the same sex, diagnosed as schizophrenic" (Fuller and Thompson, 1960, pp. 272–83; Stern, 1960, pp. 581–84).

Now the twin studies leave a good deal to be desired methodologically (Rosenthal, 1962); but there seems to be a kind of "double standard of methodological morals" in our profession, in that we place a good deal of faith in our knowledge of schizophrenic dynamics, and we make theoretical inferences about social learning factors from the establishment of group trends which may be statistically significant and replicable although of small or moderate size; but when we come to the genetic studies, our standards of rigor suddenly increase. I would argue that the concordance rates in the twin studies need not be accepted uncritically as highly precise parameter estimates in order for us to say that their magnitudes represent the most important piece of etiological information we possess about schizophrenia.

It is worthwhile, I think, to pause here over a question in the sociology of knowledge; namely, why do psychologists exhibit an aversive response to the twin data? I have no wish to argue *ad hominen* here—I raise this question in a constructive and irenic spirit because I think that a substantive confusion often lies at the bottom of this resistance, and one which can be easily dispelled. Everybody readily assents to such vague dicta as "heredity and environment interact," "there need be no conflict between organic and functional concepts," "we always deal with the total organism," and so on. But it almost seems that clinicians do not fully believe these principles in any concrete sense because they show signs of thinking that *if* a genetic basis were found for schizophrenia, the psychodynamics of the disorder (especially in relation to intrafamilial social learnings) would be somehow negated or, at least, greatly demoted in importance. To what extent, if at all, is this true?

Here we run into some widespread misconceptions as to what is meant by *specific etiology* in nonpsychiatric medicine. By postulating a "specific etiology" one does *not* imply any of the following:

1. The etiological factor always, or even usually, produces clinical illness.
2. If illness occurs, the particular form and content of symptoms are derivable by reference to the specific etiology alone.
3. The course of the illness can be materially influenced only by procedures directed against the specific etiology.
4. All persons who share the specific etiology will have closely similar histories, symptoms, and course.
5. The largest single contributor to symptom variance is the specific etiology.

In medicine, not one of these is part of the concept of specific etiology, yet they are repeatedly invoked as arguments against a genetic interpretation of schizophrenia. I am not trying to impose the causal model of medicine by analogy; I merely wish to emphasize that *if* one postulates a genetic mutation as the specific etiology of schizophrenia, he is not thereby committed to any of the above as implications. Consequently, such familiar objections as "Schizophrenics differ widely from one another" or "Many schizophrenics can be helped by purely psychological methods" should not disturb one who opts for a genetic hypothesis. In medicine, the concept of specific etiology means the *sine qua non*—the causal condition which is necessary, but not sufficient, for the disorder to occur. A genetic theory of schizophrenia would, in this sense, be stronger than that of "one contributor to variance"; but weaker than that of "largest contributor to variance." In analysis of variance terms, it means an interaction effect such that no other variables can exert a main effect when the specific etiology is lacking.

Now it goes without saying that "clinical schizophrenia" as such cannot be inherited, because it has behavioral and phenomenal contents which are learned. As Bleuler says, in order to have a delusion involving Jesuits one must first have learned about Jesuits. It seems inappropriate to apply the geneticist's concept of "penetrance" to the crude statistics of formal diagnosis—if a specific genetic etiology exists, its phenotypic expression in *psychological* categories would be a quantitative aberration in some parameter of a behavioral acquisition function. What could possibly be a genetically determined functional parameter capable of generating such diverse behavioral outcomes, including the preservation of normal function in certain domains?

The theoretical puzzle is exaggerated when we fail to conceptualize at different levels of molarity. For instance, there is a tendency among organically minded theorists to analogize between catatonic phenomena and various neurological or chemically induced states in animals. But Bleuler's masterly *Theory of Schizophrenic Negativism* (1912) shows how the whole range of catatonic behavior, including diametrically opposite modes of relating to the interpersonal environment, can be satisfactorily explained as instrumental acts; thus, even a convinced organicist, postulating a biochemical defect as specific etiology, should recognize that the causal linkage between this etiology and catatonia is indirect, requiring for the latter's derivation a lengthy chain of statements which are not even formulable except in molar psychological language.

What kind of behavioral fact about the patient leads us to diagnose schizophrenia? There are a number of traits and symptoms which get a high weight, and the weights differ among clinicians. But thought disorder continues to hold its own in spite of today's greater clinical interest in motivational (especially interpersonal) variables. If you are inclined to doubt this for yourself, consider the following indicators: Patient experiences intense ambivalence, readily reports conscious hatred of family figures, is pananxious, subjects therapist to a long series of testing operations, is withdrawn, and says, "Naturally, I am growing my father's hair."

While all of these are schizophrenic indicators, the last one is the diagnostic bell ringer. In this respect we are still Bleulerians, although we know a lot more about the schizophrenic's psychodynamics than Bleuler did. The significance of thought disorder, associative dyscontrol (or, as I prefer to call it so as to include the very mildest forms it may take, "cognitive slippage"), in schizophrenia has been somewhat deemphasized in recent years. Partly this is due to the greater interest in interpersonal dynamics, but partly also to the realization that much of our earlier psychometric assessment of the thought disorder was mainly reflecting the schizophrenic's tendency to underperform because uninterested, preoccupied, resentful, or frightened. I suggest that this realization has been overgeneralized and led us to swing too far the other way, as if we had shown that there really *is* no cognitive slippage factor present. One rather common assumption seems to be that if one can demonstrate the potentiating effect of a motivational state upon cognitive slippage, light has thereby been shed upon the etiology of schizophrenia. Why are we entitled to think this? Clinically, we see a degree of cognitive slippage not found to a comparable degree among nonschizophrenic persons. Some patients (e.g., pseudoneurotics) are highly anxious and exhibit minimal slippage; others (e.g., burnt-out cases) are minimally anxious with marked slippage. The demonstration that we can intensify a particular patient's cognitive dysfunction by manipulating his affects is not really very illuminating. After all, even ordinary neurological diseases can often be tremendously influenced symptomatically via emotional stimuli, but if a psychologist demonstrates that the spasticity or tremor of a multiple sclerotic is affected by rage or fear, we would not thereby have learned anything about the etiology of multiple sclerosis.

Consequent upon our general assimilation of the insights given us by psychoanalysis, there is today a widespread and largely unquestioned assumption that when we can trace out the motivational forces linked to the content of aberrant behavior, then we understand why the person has fallen ill. There is no compelling reason to assume this, when the evidence is mainly our dynamic understanding of the patient, however valid that may be. The phrase "why the person has fallen ill" may, of course, be legitimately taken to include these things; an account of how and when he falls ill will certainly include them. But they may be quite inadequate to answer the question, "Why does X fall ill and not Y, granted that we can understand both of them?" I like the analogy of a color psychosis, which might be developed by certain individuals in a society entirely oriented around the making of fine color discriminations. Social, sexual, economic signals are color mediated; to misuse a color word is strictly taboo; compulsive mothers are horribly ashamed of a child who is retarded in color development, and so forth. Some color-blind individuals (not all, perhaps not most) develop a color psychosis in this culture; as adults, they are found on the couches of color therapists, where a great deal of *valid* understanding is achieved about color dynamics. Some of them make a social recovery. Nonetheless, if we ask, "What was basically the matter with these patients?" meaning, "What is the specific etiology of the color psychosis?" the answer is that mutated gene on the X chromosome. This is why my own therapeutic experience with schizophrenic patients has not yet convinced me of the schizophrenogenic mother as a specific etiology, even though the picture I get of my patients' mothers is pretty much in accord with the familiar one. There is no question here of accepting the patient's account; my point is that *given* the account, and taking it quite at face value, does not tell me why the patient is a patient and not just a fellow who had a bad mother.

Another theoretical lead is the one given greatest current emphasis, namely, *interpersonal aversiveness.* The schizophrene suffers a degree of social fear, distrust, expectation of rejection and conviction of his own unlovability which cannot be matched in its depth, pervasity, and resistance to corrective experience by any other diagnostic group.

Then there is a quasi-pathognomonic sign, emphasized by Rado (1956; Rado and Daniels, 1956) but largely ignored in psychologists' diagnostic usage; namely, *anhedonia*—a marked, widespread, and refractory defect in pleasure capacity which, once you learn how to examine for it, is one of the most consistent and dramatic behavioral signs of the disease.

Finally, I include *ambivalence* from Bleuler's cardinal four (1950). His other two, "autism" and "dereism," I consider derivative from the combination of slippage, anhedonia, and aversiveness. Crudely put, if a person cannot think straight, gets little pleasure, and is afraid of everyone, he will of course learn to be autistic and dereistic.

If these clinical characterizations are correct, and we combine them with the hypothesis of a genetic specific etiology, do they give us any lead on theoretical possibilities?

Granting its initial vagueness as a construct, requiring to be filled in by neurophysiological research, I believe we should take seriously the old European notion of an "integrative neural defect" as the only direct phenotypic consequence produced by the genic mutation. This is an aberration in some parameter of single cell function, which may or may not be manifested in the functioning of more molar CNS systems, depending upon the organization of the mutual feedback controls and upon the stochastic parameters of the reinforcement regime. This neural integrative defect, which I shall christen *schizotaxia*, is all that can properly be spoken of as inherited. The imposition of a social learning history upon schizotaxic individuals results in a personality organization which I shall call, following Rado, the *schizotype.* The four core behavior traits are obviously not innate; but I postulate that they are universally learned by schizotaxic individuals, given any of the actually existing social reinforcement regimes, from the best to the worst. If the interpersonal regime is favorable, and the schizotaxic person also has the good fortune to inherit a low anxiety readiness, physical vigor, general resistance to stress and the like, he will remain a well-compensated "normal" schizotype, never manifesting symptoms of mental disease. He will be like the gout-prone male whose genes determine him to have an elevated blood uric acid titer, but who never develops clinical gout.

Only a subset of schizotypic personalities decompensate into clinical schizophrenia. It seems likely that the most important causal influence pushing the schizotype toward schizophrenic decompensation is the schizophrenogenic mother.

I hope it is clear that this view does not conflict with what has been established about the mother-child interaction. If this interaction were totally free of maternal ambivalence and aversive inputs to the schizotaxic child, even compensated schizotypy might be avoided; at most, we might expect to find only the faintest signs of cognitive slippage and other minimal neurological aberrations, possibly including body image and other proprioceptive deviations, but not the interpersonal aversiveness which is central to the clinical picture.

Nevertheless, while assuming the etiological importance of mother in determining the course of aversive social learnings, it is worthwhile to speculate about the modification our genetic equations might take on this hypothesis. Many schizophrenogenic mothers are themselves schizotypes in varying degrees of compensation. Their etiological contribution then consists jointly in their passing on the gene, *and* in the fact that being schizotypic, they provide the kind of ambivalent regime which potentiates the schizotypy of the child and raises the odds of his decompensating. Hence the incidence of the several parental genotypes among parent pairs of diagnosed proband cases is not calculable from the usual genetic formulas. For example, given a schizophrenic proband, the odds that mother is homozygous (or, if the gene were dominant, that it is mother who carries it) are different from those for father: since we have begun by selecting a decompensated case, and formal diagnosis as the phenotype involves a potentiating factor for mother which is psychodynamically greater than that for a schizotypic father. Another important influence would be the likelihood that the lower fertility of schizophrenics is also present, but to an unknown degree, among compensated schizotypes. Clinical experience suggests that in the semicompensated range, this lowering of fertility is greater among males, since many schizotypic women relate to men in an exploited or exploitive sexual way, whereas the male schizotype usually displays a marked deficit in heterosexual aggressiveness. Such a sex difference in fertility among decompensated cases has been reported by Meyers and Goldfarb (1962).

Since the extent of aversive learnings is a critical factor in decompensation, the inherited anxiety readiness is presumably greater among diagnosed cases. Since the more fertile mothers are likely to be compensated, hence themselves to be relatively low-anxiety if schizotaxic, a frequent parent pattern should be a compensated schizotypic mother married to a neurotic father, the latter being the source of the proband's high-anxiety genes (plus providing a poor paternal model for identification in male patients, and a weak defender of the child against mother's schizotypic hostility).

These considerations make ordinary family concordance studies, based upon formal diagnoses, impossible to interpret. The most important research need here is development of high-validity indicators for compensated schizotypy. I see some evidence for these conceptions in the report of Lidz and coworkers, who in studying intensively the parents of 15 schizophrenic patients were surprised to find that "minimally, 9 of the 15 patients had at least one parent who could be called schizophrenic, or ambulatory schizophrenic, or clearly paranoid in behavior and attitudes" (Lidz, Cornelison, Terry, and Fleck, 1958, p. 308). As I read the brief personality sketches presented, I would judge that all but two of the probands had a clearly schizotypic parent. These authors, while favoring a "learned irrationality" interpretation of their data, also recognize the alternative genetic interpretation. Such facts do not permit a decision obviously; my main point is the striking difference between the high incidence of parental schizotypes, mostly quite decompensated (some to the point of diagnosable psychosis), and the zero incidence which a conventional family concordance study would have yielded for this group.

Another line of evidence, based upon a very small sample but exciting because of its uniformity, is McConaghy's report (1959) that among nondiagnosed parent pairs of ten schizophrenics, subclinical thought disorder was psychometrically detectable in at least one parent of every pair. Rosenthal (1962) reports that he can add five tallies to this parent-pair count, and suggests that such results might indicate that the specific heredity is dominant, and completely penetrant, rather than recessive. The attempt to replicate these findings, and other psychometric efforts to tap subclinical cognitive slippage in the "normal" relatives of schizophrenics, should receive top priority in our research efforts.

Summarizing, I hypothesize that the statistical relation between schizotaxia, schizotypy, and schizophrenia is class inclusion: All schizotaxics become, *on all actually existing social learning regimes,* schizotypic in personality organization; but most of these remain compensated. A minority, disadvantaged by other (largely polygenically determined) constitutional weaknesses, and put on a bad regime by schizophrenogenic mothers (most of whom are themselves schizotypes) are thereby potentiated into clinical schizophrenia. What makes schizotaxia etiologically specific is its role as a *necessary* condition. I postulate that a nonschizotaxic individual, whatever his other genetic makeup and whatever his learning history, would at most develop a character disorder or a psychoneurosis; but he would not become a schizotype and therefore could never manifest its decompensated form, schizophrenia.

What sort of quantitative aberration in the structural or functional parameters of the nervous system can we conceive to be directly determined by a mutated gene, and to so alter initial dispositions that affected individuals will, in the course of their childhood learning history, develop the four schizotypal source traits: cognitive slippage, anhedonia, ambivalence, and interpersonal aversiveness? To me, the most baffling thing about the disorder is the phenotypic heterogeneity of this tetrad. If one sets himself to the task of doing a theoretical Vigotsky job on this list of psychological dispositions, he may manage part of it by invoking a sufficiently vague kind of descriptive unity between ambivalence and interpersonal aversiveness; and perhaps even anhedonia could be somehow subsumed. But the cognitive slippage presents a real roadblock. Since I consider cognitive slippage to be a core element in schizophrenia, any characterization of schizophrenic or schizotypic behavior which purports to abstract its essence but does not include the cognitive slippage must be deemed unsatisfactory. I believe that an adequate theoretical account will necessitate moving downward in the pyramid of the sciences to invoke explanatory constructs not found in social, psychodynamic, or even learning theory language, but instead at the neurophysiological level.

Perhaps we don't know enough about "how the brain works" to theorize profitably at that level; and I daresay that the more a psychologist knows about the latest research on brain function, the more reluctant he would be to engage in etiological speculation. Let me entreat my physiologically expert listeners to be charitable toward this clinician's premature speculations about how the schizotaxic brain might work. I feel partially justified in such speculating because there are some well-attested general truths about mammalian learned behavior which could almost have been set down from the armchair, in the way engineers draw block diagrams indicating what kinds of parts or subsystems a physical system *must* have, and what their interconnections *must* be, in order to function "appropriately." Brain research of the last decade provides a direct neurophysiological substrate for such cardinal behavior requirements as avoidance, escape, reward, drive differentiation, general and specific arousal or activation, and the like (Delafresnaye, 1961; Ramey and O'Doherty, 1960). The discovery in the limbic system of specific positive reinforcement centers by Olds and Milner in 1954, and of aversive centers in the same year by Delgado, Roberts, and Miller (1954), seems to me to have an importance that can scarcely be exaggerated; and while the ensuing lines of research on the laws of intracranial stimulation as a mode of behavior control present some puzzles and paradoxes, what *has* been shown up to now may already suffice to provide a theoretical framework. As a general kind of brain model let us take a broadly Hebbian conception in combination with the findings on intracranial stimulation.

To avoid repetition I shall list some basic assumptions first but introduce others in context and only implicitly when the implication is obvious. I shall assume that:

When a presynaptic cell participates in firing a postsynaptic cell, the former gains an increment in firing control over the latter. Coactivation of anatomically connected cell assemblies or assembly systems therefore increases their stochastic control linkage, and the frequency of discharges by neurons of a system may be taken as an intensity variable influencing the growth rate of intersystem control linkage as well as the momentary activity level induced in the other systems. (I shall dichotomize acquired cortical systems into "perceptual-cognitive," including central representations of goal objects; and "instrumental," including overarching monitor systems which select and guide specific effector patterns.)

Most learning in mature organisms involves altering control linkages between systems which themselves have been consolidated by previous learnings, sometimes requiring thousands of activations and not necessarily related to the reinforcement operation to the extent that perceptual-to-instrumental linkage growth functions are.

Control linkage increments from coactivation depend heavily, if not entirely, upon a period of reverberatory activity facilitating consolidation.

Feedback from positive limbic centers is facilitative to concurrent perceptual-cognitive or instrumental sequences, whereas negative center feedback exerts an inhibitory influence. (These statements refer to initial features of the direct wiring diagram, not to all long-term results of learning.) Aversive input also has excitatory effects via the arousal system, which maintain activity permitting escape learning to occur because the organism is alerted and keeps doing things. But I postulate that this overall influence is working along with an opposite effect, quite clear from both molar and intracranial experiments, that a major biological function of aversive-center activation is to produce "stoppage" of whatever the organism is currently doing.

Perceptual-cognitive systems and limbic motivational control centers develop two-way mutual controls (e.g., discriminative stimuli acquire the reinforcing property; "thoughts" become pleasantly toned; drive-relevant perceptual components are "souped-up.")

What kind of heritable parametric aberration could underlie the schizotaxic's readiness to acquire the schizotypic tetrad? It would seem, first of all, that the defect is much more likely to reside in the neurone's synaptic control function than in its storage function. It is hard to conceive of a general defect in storage which would on the one hand permit so many perceptual-cognitive functions, such as tapped by intelligence tests, school learning, or the high order cognitive powers displayed by some schizotypes, and yet have the diffuse motivational and emotional effects found in these same individuals. I am not saying that a storage deficit is clearly excludable, but it hardly seems the best place to look. So we direct our attention to parameters of control.

One possibility is to take the anhedonia as fundamental. What is *phenomenologically* a radical pleasure deficiency may be roughly identified *behaviorally* with a quantitative deficit in the positive reinforcement growth constant, and each of these—the "inner" and "outer" aspects of the organism's appetitive control system—reflect a quantitative deficit in the limbic "positive" centers. The anhedonia would then be a direct consequence of the genetic defect in wiring. Ambivalence and interpersonal aversiveness would be quantitative deviations in the balance of appetitive-aversive controls. Most perceptual-cognitive and instrumental learnings occur under mixed positive and negative schedules, so the normal consequence is a collection of habits and expectancies varying widely in the intensity of their positive and negative components, but mostly "mixed" in character. Crudely put, everybody has *some* ambivalence about almost everything, and everybody has *some* capacity for "social fear." Now, if the brain centers which mediate phenomenal pleasure and behavioral reward are numerically sparse or functionally feeble, the aversive centers meanwhile functioning normally, the long-term result would be a general shift toward the aversive end, appearing clinically as ambivalence and exaggerated interpersonal fear. If, as Brady believes, there is a wired-in reciprocal inhibiting relation between positive and negative centers, the long-term aversive drift would be further potentiated (i.e., what we see at the molar level as a sort of "softening" or "soothing" effect of feeding or petting upon anxiety elicitors would be reduced).

Cognitive slippage is not as easy to fit in, but if we assume that normal ego function is acquired by a combination of social reinforcements and the self-reinforcements which become available to the child via identification; then we might say roughly that "everybody has to learn *how* to think straight." Rationality is socially acquired; the secondary process and the reality principle are slowly and imperfectly learned, by even the most clear headed. Insofar as slippage is manifested in the social sphere, such an explanation has some plausibility. An overall aversive drift would account for the paradoxical schizotypic combination of interpersonal distortions and acute perceptiveness of others' unconscious, since the latter is really a hypersensitivity to aversive signals rather than an overall superiority in realistically discriminating social cues. On the output side, we might view the cognitive slippage of mildly schizoid speech as originating from poorly consolidated second-order "monitor" assembly systems which function in an editing role, their momentary regnancy constituting the "set to communicate." At this level, selection among competing verbal operants involves slight differences in appropriateness for which a washed-out social reinforcement history provides an insufficiently refined monitor system. However, if one is impressed with the presence of a pervasive and primary slippage, showing up in a diversity of tests (cf. Payne, 1961) and also on occasions when the patient is desperately trying to communicate, an explanation on the basis of deficient positive center activity is not too convincing.

This hypothesis has some other troubles which I shall merely indicate. Schizoid anhedonia is mainly interpersonal; i.e., schizotypes seem to derive adequate pleasure from esthetic and cognitive rewards. Secondly, some successful psychotherapeutic results include what appears to be a genuine normality of hedonic capacity. Thirdly, regressive electroshock sometimes has the same effect, and the animal evidence suggests that shock works by knocking out the aversive control system rather than by souping up appetitive centers. Finally, if the anhedonia is really general in extent, it is hard to conceive of any simple genetic basis for weakening the different positive centers, whose reactivity has been shown by Olds and others to be chemically drive specific.

A second neurological hypothesis takes the slippage factor as primary. Suppose that the immediate consequence of whatever biochemical aberration the gene directly controls were a specific alteration in the neurone's membrane stability, such that the distribution of optional transmission probabilities is more widely dispersed over the synaptic signal space than in normals. That is, presynaptic input signals whose spatio-temporal configuration locates them peripherally in the neurone's signal space yield transmission probabilities which are relatively closer to those at the maximum point, thereby producing a kind of dedifferentiation or flattening of the cell's selectivity. Under suitable parametric assumptions, this synaptic slippage would lead to a corresponding dedifferentiation of competing interassembly controls, because the elements in the less frequently or intensely coactivated control assembly would be accumulating control increments more rapidly than normal. Consider a perceptual-cognitive system whose regnancy is preponderantly associated with positive-center coactivation but sometimes with aversive. The cumulation of control increments will draw these apart; but if synaptic slippage exists, their difference, at least during intermediate stages of control development, will be attenuated. The intensity of aversive-center activation by a given level of perceptual-cognitive system activity will be exaggerated relative to that induced in the positive centers. For a preponderantly aversive control this will be reversed. But now the different algebraic sign of the feedbacks introduces an important asymmetry. Exaggerated negative feedback will tend to lower activity level in the predominantly appetitive case, retarding the growth of the control linkage, whereas exaggerated positive feedback in the predominantly aversive case will tend to heighten activity levels, accelerating the linkage growth. The long-term tendency will be that movement in the negative direction which I call *aversive drift.* In addition to the asymmetry generated by the difference in feedback signs, certain other features in the mixed-regime setup contribute to aversive drift. One factor is the characteristic difference between positive and negative reinforcers in their role as strengtheners. It seems a fairly safe generalization to say that positive centers function only weakly as strengtheners when "on" continuously, and mainly when they are turned on as terminators of a cognitive or instrumental sequence; by contrast, negative centers work mainly as "off" signals, tending to inhibit elements while steadily "on." We may suppose that the former strengthen mainly by facilitating post-activity reverberation (and hence consolidation) in successful systems, the latter mainly by holding down such reverberation in unsuccessful ones. Now, a slippage-heightened, aversive steady state during predominantly appetitive control sequences reduces their activity level, leaves fewer recently active elements available for a subsequent Olds-plus "on" signal to consolidate; whereas a slippage-heightened Olds-plus steady state during predominantly aversive control sequences (*a*) increases their negative control *during* the "on" period and (*b*) leaves relatively more of their elements recently active and hence further consolidated by the negative "off" signal when it occurs. Another factor is exaggerated competition by aversively controlled sequences, whereby the appetitive chains do not continue to the stage of receiving socially mediated positive reinforcement, because avoidant chains (e.g., phobic behavior, withdrawal, intellectualization) are getting in the way. It is worth mentioning that the schizophrenogenic mother's regime is presumably "mixed," not only in the sense of the frequent and unpredictable aversive inputs she provides in response to the child's need signals but also in her greater tendency to present such aversive inputs *concurrently* with drive reducers—thereby facilitating the "scrambling" of appetitive-and-aversive controls so typical of schizophrenia.

The schizotype's dependency guilt and aversive overreaction to offers of help are here seen as residues of the early knitting together of his cortical representations of appetitive goals with punishment-expectancy assembly systems. Roughly speaking, he has learned that to want anything interpersonally provided is to be endangered.

The cognitive slippage is here conceived as a direct molar consequence of synaptic slippage, potentiated by the disruptive effects of aversive control and inadequate development of interpersonal communication sets. Cognitive and instrumental linkages based upon sufficiently massive and consistent regimes, such as reaching for a seen pencil, will converge to asymptotes hardly distinguishable from the normal. But systems involving closely competing strengths and automatized selection among alternatives, especially when the main basis of acquisition and control is social reward, will exhibit evidences of malfunction.

My third speculative model revives a notion with a long history; namely, that the primary schizotaxic defect is a quantitative deficiency of inhibition. (In the light of Milner's revision of Hebb, in which the inhibitory action of Golgi Type II cells is crucial even for the formation of functionally differentiated cell assemblies, a defective inhibitory parameter could be an alternative basis for a kind of slippage similar in its consequences to the one we have just finished discussing.) There are two things about this somewhat moth-eaten "defective inhibition" idea which I find appealing. First, it is the most direct and uncomplicated neurologizing of the schizoid cognitive slippage. Schizoid cognitive slippage is neither an incapacity to link, nor is it an unhealthy overcapacity to link; rather, it seems to be a defective *control* over associations which are also accessible to the healthy (as in dreams, wit, psychoanalytic free association, and certain types of creative work) but are normally "edited out" or "automatically suppressed" by those superordinate monitoring assembly systems we lump together under the term "set." Secondly, in working with pseudoneurotic cases one sees a phenomenon to which insufficient theoretical attention has been paid: namely, these patients cannot turn off painful thoughts. They suffer constantly and intensely from painful thoughts about themselves, about possible adverse outcomes, about the past, about the attitudes and intentions of others. The "weak ego" of schizophrenia means a number of things, one of which is failure of defense; the schizophrenic has too ready access to his own id, and is too perceptive of the unconscious of others. It is tempting to read "failure of defense" as "quantitatively deficient inhibitory feedback." As mentioned earlier, aversive signals (whether exteroceptive or internally originated) must exert both an exciting effect via the arousal system and a quick-stoppage effect upon cortical sequences which fail to terminate the ongoing aversive signal, leading the organism to shift to another. Suppose the gene resulted in an insufficient production (or too rapid inactivation) of the specific inhibitory transmitter substance, rendering all inhibitory neurones quantitatively weaker than normal. When aversively linked cognitive sequences activate negative limbic centers, these in turn soup-up the arousal system normally but provide a subnormal inhibitory feedback, thereby permitting their elicitor to persist for a longer time and at higher intensity than normal. This further activates the negative control center, and so on, until an equilibrium level is reached which is above normal in intensity all around, and which meanwhile permits an excessive linkage growth in the aversive chain. (In this respect the semicompensated case would differ from the late-stage deteriorated schizophrenic, whose aversive drift has gradually proliferated so widely that almost any cognitive or instrumental chain elicits an overlearned defensive "stoppage," whereby even the inner life undergoes a profound and diffuse impoverishment.)

The mammalian brain is so wired that aversive signals tend to produce stoppage of regnant cognitive or instrumental sequences without the aversive signal having been specifically connected to their controlling cues or motivational systems; e.g., lever pressing under thirst or hunger can be inhibited by shock-associated buzzer, even though the latter has not been previously connected with hunger, paired with the discriminative stimulus, nor presented as punishment for the operant. A deficient capacity to inhibit concurrent activity of fringe elements (aversively connected to ambiguous social inputs from ambivalent mother) would accelerate the growth of linkages between them and appetitive systems not hitherto punished. Sequential effects are here especially important, and combine with the schizophrenogenic mother's tendency not to provide differential cues of high consistency as predictors of whether aversive or appetitive consequences will follow upon the child's indications of demand.

Consider two cortical systems having shared "fringe" subsystems (e.g., part percepts of mother's face). When exteroceptive inputs are the elicitors, negative feedback from aversive centers cannot usually produce stoppage; in the absence of such overdetermining external controls, the relative activity levels are determined by the balance of facilitative and inhibitory feedbacks. "Fringe" assemblies which have already acquired more aversive control, if they begin to be activated by regnant perceptual-cognitive sequences, will increase inhibitory feedback; and being "fringe" they can thereby be held down. The schizotaxic, whose aversive-feedback stoppage of fringe-element activity is weakened, accumulates excessive intertrial Hebbian increments toward the aversive side, the predominantly aversive fringe elements being more active and becoming more knit into the system than normally. On subsequent exteroceptively controlled trials, whenever the overdetermining stimulus input activates predominantly aversive perceptual-cognitive assemblies, their driving of the negative centers will be heightened. The resulting negative feedback may now be strong enough that, when imposed upon "fringe" assemblies weakly activated and toward the appetitive side, it can produce stoppage. On such occasions the more appetitive fringe elements will be retarded in their linkage growth, receiving fewer Hebbian increments. And those which do get over threshold will become further linked during such trials to the concurrent negative center activity. The result is twofold: a retarded growth of appetitive perceptual-cognitive linkages, and a progressive drawing of fringe elements into the aversive ambit.

"Ambiguous regimes," where the pairing of $S^+$ and $S^-$ inputs occurs very unpredictably, will have a larger number of fringe elements. Also, if the external schedule is dependent upon regnant appetitive drive states as manifested in the child's instrumental social acts, so that these are often met with mixed $S^+$ (drive-relevant) and $S^-$ (anxiety-eliciting) inputs, the appetitive and aversive assemblies will tend to become linked, and to activate positive and negative centers concurrently. The anhedonia and ambivalence would be consequences of this plus-minus "scrambling," especially if the positive and negative limbic centers are mutually inhibitory but here deficiently so. We would then expect schizotypic anhedonia to be basically interpersonal, and only derivatively present, if at all, in other contexts. This would in part explain the schizotype's preservation of relatively normal function in a large body of instrumental domains. For example, the acquisition of basic motor and cognitive skills would be relatively less geared to a mixed input, since "successful" mastery is both mechanically rewarded (e.g., how to open a door) and also interpersonally rewarded as "school success," and so forth. The hypercathexis of intellect, often found even among nonbright schizotypes, might arise from the fact that these performances are rewarded rather "impersonally" and make minimal demands on the reinforcing others. Also, the same cognitive and mechanical instrumental acts can often be employed both to turn on positive center feedback and to turn off negative, an equivalence much less true of purely social signals linked to interpersonal needs.

Having briefly sketched three neurological possibilities for postulated schizotaxic aberration, let me emphasize that while each has sufficient merit to be worth pursuing, they are mainly meant to be illustrative of the vague concept "integrative neural defect." I shall myself not be surprised if all three are refuted, whereas I shall be astounded if future research shows no fundamental aberration in nerve-cell function in the schizotype. Postulating schizotaxia as an open concept seems at first to pose a search problem of needle-in-haystack proportions, but I suggest that the plausible alternatives are really somewhat limited. After all, what does a neuron do to another neuron? It excites, or it inhibits! The schizotypic preservation of relatively normal function in selected domains directs our search toward some minimal deviation in a synaptic control parameter, as opposed to, say a gross defect in cell distribution or structure, or the kind of biochemical anomaly that yields mental deficiency. Anything which would give rise to defective storage, grossly impaired transmission, or sizable limitations on functional complexity can be pretty well excluded on present evidence. What we are looking for is a quantitative aberration in synaptic control—a deviation in amount or patterning of excitatory or inhibitory action—capable of yielding cumulative departures from normal control linkages under mixed appetitive-aversive regimes; but slight enough to permit convergence to quasi-normal asymptotes under more consistent schedules (or when massive repetition with motive-incentive factors unimportant is the chief basis for consolidation). The defect must generate aversive drift on mixed social reinforcement regimes, and must yield a primary cognitive slippage which, however, may be extremely small in magnitude except as potentiated by the cumulative effects of aversive drift. Taken together these molar constraints limit our degrees of freedom considerably when it comes to filling in the neurophysiology of schizotaxia.

Leaving aside the specific nature of schizotaxia, we must now raise the familiar question whether such a basic neurological defect, however subtle and nonstructural it might be, should not have been demonstrated hitherto? In reply to this objection I shall content myself with pointing out that there are several lines of evidence which, while not strongly arguing *for* a neurological theory, are rebuttals of an argument presupposing clear and consistent *negative* findings. For example: Ignoring several early European reports with inadequate controls, the literature contains a half-dozen quantitative studies showing marked vestibular system dysfunction in schizophrenics (Angyal and Blackman, 1940, 1941; Angyal and Sherman, 1942; Colbert and Koegler, 1959; Freedam and Rodnick, 1942; Leach, 1960; Payne and Hewlett, 1960; Pollock and Krieger, 1958). Hoskins (1946) concluded that a neurological defect in the vestibular system was one of the few clear-cut biological findings in the Worcester studies. It is of prime importance to replicate these findings among compensated and pseudoneurotic cases, where the diffuse withdrawal and deactivation factor would not provide the explanation it does in the chronic, burnt-out case (cf. Collins, Crampton, and Posner, 1961). Another line of evidence is in the work of King (1954) on psychomotor deficit, noteworthy for its careful use of task simplicity, asymptote performance, concern for patient cooperation, and inclusion of an outpatient pseudoneurotic sample. King himself regards his data as indicative of a rather basic behavior defect, although he does not hold it to be schizophrenia-specific. Then we have such research as that of Barbara Fish (1961), indicating the occurrence of varying signs of perceptual-motor maldevelopment among infants and children who subsequently manifest clinical schizophrenia. The earlier work of Schilder and Bender along these lines is, of course, well known, and there has always been a strong minority report in clinical psychiatry that many schizophrenics provide subtle and fluctuating neurological signs of the "soft" variety, if one keeps alert to notice or elicit them. I have myself been struck by the frequent occurrence, even among pseudoneurotic patients, of transitory neurologic-like complaints (e.g., diplopia, localized weakness, one-sided tremor, temperature dyscontrol, dizziness, disorientation) which seem to lack dynamic meaning or secondary gain and whose main effect upon the patient is to produce bafflement and anxiety. I have seen preliminary findings by J. McVicker Hunt and his students in which a rather dramatic quantitative deficiency in spatial cognizing is detectable in schizophrenics of above-normal verbal intelligence. Research by Cleveland (1960; Cleveland, Fisher, Reitman, and Rothaus, 1962) and by Arnhoff and Damianopoulos (1964) on the clinically well-known body-image anomalies in schizophrenia suggests that this domain yields quantitative departures from the norm of such magnitude that with further instrumental and statistical refinement it might be used as a quasi-pathognomonic sign of the disease. It is interesting to note a certain thread of unity running through this evidence, which perhaps lends support to Rado's hypothesis that a kinesthetic integrative defect is even more characteristic of schizotypy than is the radical anhedonia.

All these kinds of data are capable of a psychodynamic interpretation. "Soft" neurological signs are admittedly ambiguous, especially when found in the severely decompensated case. The only point I wish to make here is that *since* they exist and are at present unclear in etiology, an otherwise plausible neurological view cannot be refuted on the ground that there is a *lack* of any sign of neurological dysfunction in schizophrenia; there is no such lack.

Time forces me to leave detailed research strategy for another place, but the main directions are obvious and may be stated briefly: The clinician's Mental Status ratings on anhedonia, ambivalence, and interpersonal aversiveness should be objectified and preferably replaced by psychometric measures. The research findings on cognitive slippage, psychomotor dyscontrol, vestibular malfunction, body image, and other spatial aberrations should be thoroughly replicated and extended into the pseudoneurotic and semicompensated ranges. If these efforts succeed, it will be possible to set up a multiple sign pattern, using optimal cuts on phenotypically diverse indicators, for identifying compensated schizotypes in the nonclinical population. Statistics used must be appropriate to the theoretical model of a dichotomous latent taxonomy reflecting itself in otherwise independent quantitative indicators. Family concordance studies should then be run, relating proband schizophrenia to schizotypy as identified by this multiple indicator pattern. Meanwhile, we should carry on an active and varied search for more direct neurological signs of schizotaxia, concentrating our hunches on novel stimulus inputs (for example, the stabilized retinal image situation) that may provide a better context for basic neural dysfunction to show up—instead of being masked by learned compensations or imitated by psychopathology.

In closing, I should like to take this unusual propaganda opportunity to play the prophet. It is my strong personal conviction that such a research strategy will enable psychologists to make a unique contribution in the near future, using psychological techniques to establish that schizophrenia, while its content is learned, is fundamentally a neurological disease of genetic origin.

## REFERENCES


Angyal, A., and N. Blackman, "Vestibular Reactivity in Schizophrenia," *Arch. Neurol. Psychiat.*, 44 (1940), 611–20.

Angyal, A., and N. Blackman, "Paradoxical Reactions in Schizophrenia Under the Influence of Alcohol, Hyperpnea, and $CO_2$ Inhalation," *Amer. J. Psychiat.*, 97 (1941), 893–903.

Angyal, A., and N. Sherman, "Postular Reactions to Vestibular Stimulation in Schizophrenic and Normal Subjects," *Amer. J. Psychiat.*, 98 (1942), 857–62.

Arnhoff, F., and E. Damianopoulos, "Self-body Recognition in Schizophrenia," *J. Genet. Psychol.*, 70 (1964), 353–61.

Bleuler, E., *Theory of Schizophrenic Negativism* (New York: Nervous and Mental Disease Publishing Company, 1912).

Bleuler, E., *Dementia Praecox* (New York: International Universities Press, 1950).

Cleveland, S. E., "Judgment of Body Size in a Schizophrenic and a Control Group," *Psychol. Rep.*, 7 (1960), 304.

Cleveland, S. E., S. Fisher, E. E. Reitman, and P. Rothaus, "Perception of Body Size in Schizophrenia," *Arch. Gen. Psychiat.*, 7 (1962), 277–85.

Colbert, G. and R. Koegler, "Vestibular Dysfunction in Childhood Schizophrenia," *AMA Arch. Gen. Psychiat.*, 1 (1959), 600–17.

Collins, W. E., G. H. Crampton, and J. B. Posner, "The Effect of Mental Set upon Vestibular Nystagmus and the EEG," *USA Med. Res. Lab. Rep.*, No. 439 (1961).

Delafresnaye, J. F., ed., *Brain Mechanisms and Learning* (Springfield, Illinois: Charles C Thomas, 1961).

Delgado, J. M. R., W. W. Roberts, and N. E. Miller, "Learning Motivated by Electrical Stimulation of the Brain," *Amer. J. Physiol.*, 179 (1954), 587–93.

Fish, Barbara, "The Study of Motor Development in Infancy and Its Relationship to Psychological Functioning," *Amer. J. Psychiat.*, 117 (1961), 1113–18.

Freedam, H., and E. H. Rodnick, "Effect of Rotation on Postural Steadiness in Normal and Schizophrenic Subjects," *Arch. Neurol. Psychiat.*, 48 (1942)), 47–53.

Fuller, J. L., and W. R. Thompson, *Behavior Genetics* (New York: John Wiley, 1960), pp. 272–83.

Hoskins, R. G., *The Biology of Schizophrenia* (New York: W. W. Norton, 1946).

King, H. E., *Psychomotor Aspects of Mental Disease* (Cambridge: Harvard University Press, 1954).

Leach, W. W., "Nystagmus: An Integrative Neural Deficit in Schizophrenia," *J. Abnorm. Soc. Psychol.*, 60 (1960), 305–309.

Lidz, T., A. Cornelison, D. Terry, and S. Fleck, "Intrafamilial Environment of the Schizophrenic Patient: VI. The Transmission of Irrationality," *AMA Arch. Neurol. Psychiat.*, 79 (1958), 305–16.

McConaghy, N., "The Use of an Object Sorting Test in Elucidating the Hereditary Factor in Schizophrenia," *J. Neurol. Neurosurg. Psychiat.*, 22 (1959), 243–46.

Meyers, D., and W. Goldfarb, "Psychiatric Appraisals of Parents and Siblings of Schizophrenic Children," *Amer. J. Psychiat.*, 118 (1962), 902–908.

Olds, J., and P. Milner, "Positive Reinforcement Produced by Electrical Stimulation of Septal Area and Other Regions of Rat Brain," *J. Comp. Physiol. Psychol.*, 47 (1954), 419–27.

Payne, R. W., "Cognitive Abnormalities," in H. J. Eysenck, ed., *Handbook of Abnormal Psychology* (New York: Basic Books, 1961), pp. 248–50.

Payne, R. S., and J. H. G. Hewlett, "Thought Disorder in Psychotic Patients," in H. J. Eysenck, ed., *Experiments in Personality* (vol. 2; London: Routledge & Kegan Paul, 1960), pp. 3–106.

Pollack, M., and H. P. Krieger, "Oculomotor and Postural Patterns in Schizophrenic Children," *AMA Arch. Neurol. Psychiat.*, 79 (1958), 720–26.

Rado, S., *Psychoanalysis of Behavior* (New York: Grune and Stratton, 1956).

Rado, S., and G. Daniels, *Changing Concepts of Psychoanalytic Medicine* (New York: Grune and Stratton, 1956).

Ramey, E. R., and D. S. O'Doherty, eds., *Electrical Studies on the Unanesthetized Brain* (New York: Hoeber, 1960).

Rosenthal, D., "Problems of Sampling and Diagnosis in the Major Twin Studies of Schizophrenia," *J. Psychiat. Res.*, 1 (1962) 116–34.

Stern, K., *Principles of Human Genetics* (San Francisco: Freeman, 1960), pp. 581–84.

# 2 : Disorders of Attention and Perception in Early Schizophrenia

ANDREW McGHIE
JAMES CHAPMAN

Our main purpose here is to trace the development of a hypothesis relating to early schizophrenia and to outline a proposed method of investigation to test the validity of the theory advanced. In an earlier study of the chronic schizophrenic condition (Freeman, Cameron and McGhie, 1958), an attempt was made to outline a comprehensive theory which would account for the diverse pathological behaviour of chronic schizophrenic patients. Although this investigation was psychoanalytic in orientation, in its conceptual framework leaning heavily on Federn's (1953) theoretical model of the psychosis, the authors' observations led them to reject the proposal that schizophrenic symptoms are defensive activities purposefully related to unconscious conflicts over interpersonal difficulties. The basic pathological breakdown was observed to lie in an

Reprinted by permission of the authors and publisher from *British Journal of Medical Psychology*, 34 (1961), 103–17. The authors acknowledge "the advice and encouragement given by Dr. I. R. C. Batchelor, Physician Superintendent, Dundee Royal Mental Hospital."

impairment of ego functions, particularly in the process of perception. It seemed to the authors that it would be more accurate to describe the process in reverse, arguing that the breakdown in interpersonal difficulties was a reaction to the primary cognitive disturbance. A comparison of the chronic schizophrenic patient's behaviour with that of the young child (Freeman and McGhie, 1957) substantiated this view that the basic disturbance in schizophrenia was a cognitive one which caused the patient to operate at a perceptual level comparable to the primitive and unorganized processes characteristic of infancy and childhood.

Such observations are limited by the relative inability of the chronic patient to communicate directly and to describe his subjective experiences in a comprehensive manner. Although it might be argued that the relative inacessibility of the chronic schizophrenic patient is an essential part of the disease process, it is very likely that it is also partially an artifact produced by prolonged hospitalization. In view of this, attention was turned to schizophrenic patients who could be observed at an early stage of their psychotic illness. One of the present authors (Chapman) examined a few of these early patients over a period of time in a psychotherapeutic setting, and the clinical material which emerged in one of these cases was discussed in a later paper (Chapman, Freeman, and McGhie, 1959). Such observations of a few early schizophrenic patients during psychotherapy endorsed the opinion that the fundamental disorder in schizophrenia was a cognitive one, most clearly evident in the fields of attention and perception, and that other aspects of the patient's symptomatology could be interpreted as his reactions to this basic disorder. It was also felt that a study of the early schizophrenic patient was much more rewarding in that the primary impairments were accessible to study, being unobscured by secondary reactions that occur in the later stages of the illness.

While the primary cognitive disturbance had earlier been described in terms of a breakdown of ego structure, it seemed to the present authors that this theoretical framework was now too narrow, particularly in that it did not easily allow a theoretical *rapprochement* with work in other related fields. In continuing the clinical study on early schizophrenic patients, the orientation was changed, not only to accentuate the patient's current mental activities but also so that cognitive disturbances would constitute the main field of inquiry. A standard method of interviewing patients along these lines was drawn up and subsequently applied in a clinical study of early schizophrenic patients. The interview concentrated on recent changes in the patients' experiences and encouraged them to describe these changes in their own words. The clinical material was collected under categories which reflected the main areas of cognitive function. The most useful arrangement of categories was found to include the processes of attention, perception, motility, and thinking. Attention was also paid to changes in affect which were observable. A total of twenty-six early schizophrenic patients, where the subsequent course of the illness confirmed the original diagnosis, were examined in this way, and this report will deal mainly with the analysis of the clinical material so gathered, leading to a hypothesis regarding the nature of the primary disorder in schizophrenia.

The interviews were not carried out in a formal setting, the patient merely being encouraged to speak about his present difficulties and his speech recorded in the form of verbatim notes. In order to cover the full range of topics contained in the standard interview, it was necessary to see most of the patients concerned on several occasions, the total interviewing time for patients ranging thus from two to twelve hours.

## Clinical Material

The interview material was analysed by breaking it up into a number of separate statements, each representing the patient's description of a symptomatic alteration in his experience. These separate statements were then arranged by the authors in categories which appeared to them to agree with the form and direction of the symptom being described. The small numbers in the group being studied obviously preclude any statistical analysis. As it is equally impossible to give a detailed description of each patient's account, the procedure here has been to give in each category a sample of the verbatim statements made by patients, which appear to the authors to have such a high incidence of frequency as to allow them to be considered as representative of the group as a whole. As will be apparent, the assigning of many of these statements to different categories is to some extent arbitrary in that the patients' comments are at times equally relevant to two or more categories at the same time. This is of course not surprising, the categories representing divisions of the cognitive field which are in themselves artificial, although useful for the purposes of analysis. Each statement reported here is prefaced by the patient's number in the group, this being done mainly to avoid the necessity of introducing each statement in turn.

### *1. Disturbances in the Process of Attention*

*Patient* 11. It's as if I am too wide awake—very, very alert. I can't relax at all. Everything seems to go through me. I just can't shut things out.

*Patient* 5. I listen to sounds all the time. I let all the sounds come in that are there. I should really get an earphone and a wireless and control these sounds coming in so that at least I know they are separate from me.

*Patient* 13. My concentration is very poor. I jump from one thing to another. If I am talking to someone they only need to cross their legs or scratch their heads and I am distracted and forget what I was saying. I think I could concentrate better with my eyes shut.

*Patient* 14. Things are coming in too fast. I lose my grip

of it and get lost. I am attending to everything at once and as a result I do not really attend to anything.

*Patient* 2. I can't concentrate. It's diversion of attention that troubles me. I am picking up different conversations. It's like being a transmitter. The sounds are coming through to me but I feel my mind cannot cope with everything. It's difficult to concentrate on any one sound. It's like trying to do two or three different things at the one time.

*Patient* 23. Everything seems to grip my attention although I am not particularly interested in anything. I am speaking to you just now but I can hear noises going on next door and in the corridor. I find it difficult to shut these out and it makes it more difficult for me to concentrate on what I am saying to you. Often the silliest little things that are going on seem to interest me. That's not even true; they don't interest me but I find myself attending to them and wasting a lot of time this way. I know that sounds like laziness but it's not really.

*Patient* 7. Everything that's going on seems to be picked up by me, almost as if I welcome these things to stop me attending fully to any one thing.

*Patient* 6. I am easily put off what I am doing or even what I am talking about. If something else is going on somewhere, even just a noise, it interrupts my thoughts and they get lost. If I am somewhere where there is a lot going on I am swinging from one thing to another instead of concentrating on one thing and getting it done.

*Patient* 25. I can't concentrate on television because I can't watch the screen and listen to what is being said at the same time. I can't seem to take in two things like this at the same time, especially when one of them means watching and the other means listening. On the other hand I seem to be always taking in too much at the one time and then I can't handle it and can't make sense of it.

The implications of these comments will be considered in detail after we have examined the clinical material as a whole.

One might, however, at this point note that the reports in this section appear to be related to a general factor of distractibility. These patients appear to have lost the ability and freedom to direct their attention *focally,* as required in normal concentration. Their attention is instead directed *radially* in a manner which is determined, not by the individual's volition, but by the diffuse pattern of stimuli existing in the total environmental situation. In effect, what seems to be happening is that the individual finds himself less free to direct his attention at will. Instead, his control of attention is now being increasingly determined for him by concrete changes in the environment. To this extent, the patient feels "open," vulnerable, and in danger of having his personal identity swamped by the incoming tide of impressions which he cannot control.

## *2. Disturbances in the Process of Perception*

### A. CHANGES IN SENSORY QUALITY

*Patient* 2. During the last while back I have noticed that noises all seem to be louder to me than they were before. It's as if someone had turned up the volume. . . . I notice it most with background noises—you know what I mean, noises that are always around but you don't notice them. Now they seem to be just as loud and sometimes louder than the main noises that are going on. . . . It's a bit alarming at times because it makes it difficult to keep your mind on something when there's so much going on that you can't help listening to.

*Patient* 17. Colors seem to be brighter now, almost as if they are luminous. When I look around me it's like a luminous painting. I'm not sure if things are solid until I touch them.

*Patient* 23. Sometimes I feel all right then the next minute I feel that everything is coming towards me. I see things more than what they really are. Everything's brighter and louder and noisier.

*Patient* 15. I seem to be noticing colors more than before, although I am not artistically minded. The colors of things seem much more clearer and yet at the same time there is something missing. The things I look at seem to be flatter, as if you were looking just at a surface. Maybe it's because I notice so much more about things and find myself looking at them for a longer time. Not only the color of things fascinates me but all sorts of little things, like markings in the surface, pick up my attention too.

*Patient* 11. I have noticed a lot recently that I seem to get a little mixed up about where sounds are coming from. Often I have to check up if someone speaks to me and several times I thought someone was shouting through the window when it was really the wireless at the front of the house.

*Patient* 18. I've had difficulty in tracing where sounds are coming from, although I am not deaf. If the wireless is on, for example, I know the wireless is there but sometimes I feel that the sounds are coming from behind my back.

*Patient* 10. Have you ever had wax in your ears for a while and then had them syringed? That's what it's like now, as if I had been deaf before. Everything is much noisier and it excites me.

### B. PERCEPTION OF SPEECH

*Patient* 5. When people are talking I have to think what the words mean. You see, there is an interval instead of a spontaneous response. I have to think about it and it takes time. I have to pay all my attention to people when they are speaking or I get all mixed up and don't understand them.

*Patient* 18. If there are three or four people talking at one time I can't take it in. I would not be able to hear what they were saying properly and I would get the one mixed up with the other. To me it's just like a babble—a noise that goes right through me.

*Patient* 22. When people are talking I just get scraps of it. If it is just one person who is speaking that's not so bad, but if others join in, then I can't pick it up at all. I just can't get into tune with that conversation. It makes me feel open—as if things are closing in on me and I have lost control.

*Patient* 15. It's the same with listening. You only hear snatches of conversation and you can't fit them together.

*Patient* 9. Sometimes when people speak to me my head is overloaded. It's too much to hold at once. It goes out as quick as it goes in. It makes you forget what you just heard because you can't get hearing it long enough. It's just words in the air unless you can figure it out from their faces.

*Patient* 3. When people are talking the words are going on and on and I don't understand them. It's extremely confusing—like going into a blank wall.

*Patient* 12. I'm slow in everything and everything is too quick. People speak to me but they go too quick for me to pick up. It's not that they talk too fast; it's me that's slow.

*Patient* 19. I can concentrate quite well on what people are saying if they talk simply. It's when they go into long sentences that I lose the meanings. It just becomes a lot of words that I would need to string together to make sense.

*Patient* 6. I'm a good listener but often I'm not really taking it in. I nod my head and smile but it's just a lot of jumbled up words to me.

### C. PERCEPTION AND MOVEMENT

*Patient* 7. I can't move if I am distracted by too much noise. I can't help stopping to listen. That's what happens when I am lying in bed. If there's too much noise going on I can't move.

*Patient* 12. I get stuck, almost as if I am paralysed at times. It may only last for a minute or two but it's a bit frightening. It seems to happen even when something unexpected takes place, especially if there's a lot of noise that comes on suddenly. Say I am walking across the floor and someone suddenly switches on the wireless; the music seems to stop me in my tracks and sometimes I freeze like that for a minute or two.

*Patient* 22. Sounds sometimes make me feel dizzy. If I am

looking at something and there's a sudden noise, perhaps an airplane passing or a bus, what I am looking at seems to swing or move in front of me, although I know it's stationary. It makes me feel giddy but it does not last for long.

*Patient* 3. Everything is in bits. You put the picture up bit by bit into your head. It's like a photograph that's torn in bits and put together again. You have to absorb it again. If you move it's frightening. The picture you had in your head is still there but it's broken up. If I move there's a new picture that I have to put together again.

*Patient* 5. My responses are too slow. Things happen too quickly. There's too much to take in and I try to take in everything. Things happen but I don't respond. When something happens quickly or unexpectedly it stuns me like a shock. I just get stuck. I've got to be prepared and ready for such things. Nothing must come upon me too quickly.

*Patient* 20. When I have been rushing about I have to stop and be still for a minute. It's like watching a miniature railway. There is split second timing. One train misses the other by a split second. If I could walk slowly I would get on all right. My brain is going too quickly. If I move quickly I don't take things in. My brain is working all right but I am not responding to what is coming into it. My mind is always taking in little things at the side.

*Patient* 14. I don't like moving fast. I feel there would be a breakup if I went too quick. I can only stand that a short time and then I have to stop. If I carried on I wouldn't be aware of things as they really are. I would just be aware of the sound and the noise and the movements. Everything would be a jumbled mass. I have found that I can stop this happening by going completely still and motionless. When I do that, things are easier to take in.

*Patient* 1. When I move quickly it's a strain on me. Things go too quick for my mind. They get blurred and it's like being blind. It's as if you were seeing a picture one moment and another picture the next. I just stop and watch my feet. Everything is all right if I stop, but if I start moving again I lose control.

The first type of perceptual change reported by the patients appears as a heightening of sensory vividness which is experienced particularly in the auditory and visual fields. These subjective experiences might be interpreted as a further extension of the loss in the selective function of attention as suggested in the previous section. In normal perception we are aware of only a small but significant sector of the total field of sensory stimulation. The reports here indicate that the patients find themselves attending, in an involuntary fashion, to features of their perceptual field which have hitherto occupied a background position. This widening of the range of conscious perception tends to disturb the constancy and stability of the perceptual matrix, thus causing a changing sense of subjective reality.

The second category of perceptual change is related to a disturbance in the perception of speech patterns. In normal communication incoming information is identified and fitted into context automatically, without the need of conscious intervention. Words are perceived, not as such, but as part of a total pattern of communication following a specific theme which contains a positive sense of direction in its elaboration. This automatic ordering of the separate items of verbal communication into a meaningful sequence leaves the individual free to concentrate on the development of the theme rather than on its construction. From the reports given here it would seem that the patients are unable to appreciate the *content* of the communication because their conscious attention is taken up by the *form*. Their perceptual system is indeed overloaded and, unless enough time is allowed for both the form and content of the communication to be consciously assessed, effective registration does not take place. This dysfunction might be seen as related to the phenomenon of sensory vividness already discussed, in that both changes in experience result from the emergence into conscious awareness of perceptual features which have hitherto functioned autonomously.

In the third category of perceptual experience reported, the patients appear to be describing brief catatonic episodes which are causally related to changes in the auditory and visual fields. The production of a response in one sense modality by the stimulation of another sense modality was noted earlier in a study of chronic schizophrenic patients (Freeman and McGhie, 1957), and was also reported in a detailed study of a young patient (Chapman *et al.*, 1959). This type of perceptual fusion, similar to synaesthesia, is the basis of Werner and Wapner's concept of "functional equivalence," which they found to be present in the behaviour of young children. In their experiments it was found that both auditory and tactile stimulation led to an identical perceptual change in the visual field. The descriptions given by the patients also correspond with Piaget's (1951) studies of early perceptual development in childhood when the slightest alteration in the perceptual field results in the whole structure of that field being altered. In this primitive and undifferentiated state motility and perception are intimately linked, motility being dependent upon stability of the perceptual field. The same process would seem to lie behind the difficulties of these early schizophrenic patients who declare, "Everything is all right if I stop, but if I start moving again I lose control." The early schizophrenic patient thus demonstrates in his reactions a pronounced degree of diffuseness between normally discrete sensory channels and a lack of stability in perception. Once again we see the young schizophrenic patient finding himself faced with a new unstable and fluctuating relationship with his environment in which he no longer exerts the initiative.

### *3. Changes in Motility and Bodily Awareness*

*Patient* 18. I am not sure of my own movements any more. It's very hard to describe this but at times I am not sure about even simple actions like sitting down. It's not so much thinking out what to do, it's the doing of it that sticks me. . . . I found recently that I was thinking of myself doing things before I would do them. If I am going to sit down, for example, I have got to think of myself and almost see myself sitting down before I do it. It's the same with other things like washing, eating and even dressing—things that I have done at one time without even bothering or thinking about at all. . . . All this makes me move much slower now. I take more time to do things because I am always conscious of what I am doing. If I could just stop noticing what I am doing, I would get things done a lot faster.

*Patient* 11. You see, I've got to think ahead before rushing into something. If I went straight ahead I might fall down or something. I've got to see that the path is clear.

*Patient* 12. If you move fast without thinking, co-ordination becomes difficult and everything becomes mechanical. I prefer to think out movements first before I do anything; then I get up slowly and do it.

*Patient* 23. People just do things but I have to watch first to see how you do things. I have to think out most things first and know how to do them before I do them. When I am racing and am ready to get off the mark I have to think of putting my hands down in front of me and how to lift my legs before I can start.

*Patient* 19. I have got to see ahead. I keep to a pattern. If you rush you might do things wrong. If people rush at things their minds are probably away somewhere else anyway, but I know what's happening all the time.

*Patient* 7. Anticipation is one of my worst habits. I have to think of what I am going to do all the time and that takes up a lot of energy and when I am doing something I am aware of my every movement.

*Patient* 14. If I am doing something, then I start thinking of what I am doing; that locks me up in a sense. For example, if I drop something and stop to pick it up, if I start to think of myself in that position and what I am doing, that locks me up in that position. If you keep thinking of where your body is it gets locked up.

*Patient* 3. I have to do everything step by step, nothing is automatic now. Everything has to be considered.

*Patient* 17. People go about completely unthinking. They do things automatically. A man can walk down the street and not bother. If he stops to think about it he might look at his legs and just wonder where he is going to get the energy to move his legs. His legs will start to wobble. How does he know that his legs are going to move when he wants them to?

One of the most important features of normal motility is our ability to initiate and carry out sequences of motor response without conscious deliberation. Through repetition we gradually build up a store of activities, simple and complex, which require only an awareness of an end goal to reproduce the activity in a spontaneous and skilled manner. Without this automatic regulative function, normal behaviour would be hopelessly complex, requiring conscious coordination of every simple sequence of movement. The descriptions of these patients indicate a loss of this spontaneity caused by a heightened awareness of the bodily sensations and volitional impulses normally lying outside of conscious experience. Each action now has to be planned and executed step by step with a great deal of conscious deliberation. The patient finds himself becoming increasingly "self-conscious" in an entirely literal sense.

### *4. Changes in the Process of Thinking*

*Patient* 9. My thoughts get all jumbled up. I start thinking or talking about something but I never get there. Instead I wander off in the wrong direction and get caught up with all sorts of different things that may be connected with the things I want to say but in a way I can't explain. People listening to me get more lost than I do.

*Patient* 20. My trouble is that I've got too many thoughts. You might think about something—let's say that ashtray—and just think, oh yes, that's for putting my cigarette in, but I would think of it and then I would think of a dozen different things connected with it at the same time.

*Patient* 21. My mind's away. I have lost control. There are too many things coming into my head at once and I can't sort them out.

*Patient* 6. My mind is going too quick for me. It is all bamboozled. All the things are going too quick for me. Everything's too fast and too big for me.

*Patient* 15. It's not that I can't concentrate right, it's just that I can't concentrate on the major issues. I get fogged up with all the different bits and lose the important things in the picture. I find myself paying attention to all sorts of tiny things instead of getting on with the things I should be doing. I have to concentrate on simple things like walking, peddling my bike, and even talking.

*Patient* 22. I let my mind wander for a minute but sometimes for half an hour. I just go into myself. I just stop moving. I may be looking at something in a window, for example, and then I find myself thinking deeper and getting caught up in it. My mind can't move past it. When I come to, I find I have been just thinking about the one thing for a long time and I panic, and then I start to worry if people have seen me.

*Patient* 4. I may be thinking quite clearly and telling someone something and suddenly I get stuck. You have seen me do this and you may think I am just lost for words or that I have gone into a trance, but that is not what happens. What happens is that I suddenly stick on a word or an idea in my head and I just can't move past it. It seems to fill my mind and there's no room for anything else. This might go on for a while and suddenly it's over. Afterwards I get a feeling that I have been thinking very deeply about whatever it was but often I can't remember what it was that has filled my mind so completely.

*Patient* 13. If I am reading I may suddenly get bogged down at a word. It may be any word, even a simple word that I know well. When this happens I can't get past it. It's as if

I am being hypnotized by it. It's as if I am seeing the word for the first time and in a different way from anyone else. It's not so much that I absorb it, it's more like it absorbing me.

*Patient* 18. I just can't concentrate on anything. There's too much going on in my head and I can't sort it out. My thoughts wander round in circles without getting anywhere. I try to read even a paragraph in a book but it takes me ages because each bit I read starts me thinking in ten different directions at once.

*Patient* 2. When I am trying to think of something I am like a railway engine running along a line where someone keeps changing the points.

*Patient* 4. It's either one extreme or the other with me. Sometimes I can't concentrate because my brain is going too fast and at other times it is either going too slow or has stopped altogether. I don't mean that my mind becomes a blank; it just gets stuck in a rut when I am thinking over and over again about one thing. It's just as if there was a crack in the record.

Normal thinking involves the purposeful manipulation of the internal images and ideas that form our stock of previously acquired information. In bringing our thoughts to bear on a specific problem, we abstract from the total field of information that which is relevant to the task in hand. Thinking—or, more accurately, reasoning—is thus a highly selective process in which inhibition is intimately linked with the degree of abstractness of the thought product. Indeed, the concept of control, direction, and inhibition is central to the process of logical reasoning. In conditions of relaxed control, such as in the hypnagogic state and in sleep, our thinking loses this sense of direction and is no longer oriented towards reality. Logical sequences of ideas are replaced by merely associative sequences, and the thought level passes from the abstract to the concrete. It is this very lack of control, direction, and inhibition which characterizes the disturbances of thinking reported by our patients. As one of the patients put it during interview: "I wish I could think without interruption—not from others but from inside myself."

## *5. Changes in the Affective Process*

*Patient* 2. You have no idea what it's like, Doctor. You would have to experience it yourself. When you feel yourself going into a sort of coma you get really scared. It's like waiting on a landing craft going into D-Day. You tremble and panic. It's like no other fear on earth.

*Patient* 7. When I am walking along the street it comes on me. I start to think deeply and I start to go into a trance. I think so deep that I almost get out of this world. Then you get frightened that you are going to get into a jam and lose yourself. That's when I get worried and excited.

*Patient* 21. Things just happen to me now and I have no control over them. I don't seem to have the same say in things any more. At times I can't even control what I want to think about. I am starting to feel pretty numb about everything because I am becoming an object and objects don't have feelings.

*Patient* 19. Half the time I am talking about one thing and thinking about half a dozen other things at the same time. It must look queer to people when I laugh about something that has got nothing to do with what I am talking about, but they don't know what's going on inside and how much of it is running round in my head. You see, I might be talking about something quite serious to you and other things come into my head at the same time that are funny and this makes me laugh. If I could only concentrate on the one thing at the one time I wouldn't look half so silly.

*Patient* 14. It's just that I seem to be changing and I can't do anything about it. I feel I am losing myself more each day. That's bad enough but it's the vagueness of the whole thing that really troubles me. If the things that were happening were clearer so you could put them into words and tell somebody what it's like without sounding quite daft, it wouldn't be so bad.

The comments made by the patients suggest that the affective changes reported are causally related to the cognitive changes which we have already described. These patients (e.g., patients 2 and 7) first react with perplexity, anxiety, and panic to the pathological changes in their experience into which, at this stage of their illness, they have a fair degree of insight. Later, as they find themselves gradually losing control over cognitive and volitional activities, the mental and bodily ego is experienced as increasingly alien (patients 21, 19, and 14). Losing their subjectivity, they are becoming objects and, as one patient said, "Objects don't have feelings." The main point we would wish to make here, however, is that when these affective changes are reported they would appear to be secondary and to follow as reactions to the patient's awareness of the primary cognitive changes which have already taken place.

## Discussion

Studies of early ego development, particularly those by genetic psychologists such as Piaget and Werner, indicate that the first stages of infancy are characterized by an undifferentiated protoplasmic consciousness in which there is no differentation between the self and the outside world; no self-awareness; no consciousness of external objects. This stage of adualism, which approximates to the Freudian concept of an undifferentiated ego-id, is gradually superseded by the individuation of the developing ego. In these early stages of infancy it would appear that the infant passively assimilates or incorporates mental experiences in an undiscriminated fashion, whether these experiences originate externally from the environment or internally within the infant's own body. The process of perception at this time is primitive, global, and undifferentiated, the infant having virtually no control over the mass of incoming sensory stimuli reaching his primitive nervous system. In its subsequent development the ego must gain an increasing degree of mastery over its environment by controlling and organizing the incoming flow of sensory stimuli. For this to take place, we must postulate an internal mechanism which allows the organism to select from this diffuse sensory input the information necessary to allow it to function efficiently. To a large extent, adjustment to the environment, and the development of a differentiated ego, develops by a process of selection and inhibition of incoming sensory stimuli, so that only part of the whole sensory background is effectively registered in consciousness.

It is perhaps well if we pause at this point to define in more detail our use of the word "consciousness." In examining the variety of meanings given to the term in the symposium, *Brain Mechanisms and Consciousness* (1954), Brain (1958) finds that the term may be used to mean at least six different things. Among the definitions of consciousness given in the Symposium to which Brain referred we might select the following statement by Jung (1954) as being nearest to our own interpretation: "Consciousness is considered as a selective and restraining function for limiting actual psychic experience amongst the many potentially psychic phenomena which remain unconscious. Attention is a coordinating aid for conscious perception and may be compared to a spotlight which illuminates details in the dark, unconscious field of the internal and external world. . . . Attention assists consciousness by selecting inner experience and outer perceptions from the sense organs, so illuminating a section of the internal and external world." By the process of attention we thus break down and effectively categorise both the information reaching us from the environment and that which is internally available in the form of stored past experience. It would seem that in the earlier stages of development, consciousness consists merely of a passive assimilation of sensations, and that perception is then dependent upon each change in the sensory input. We have already referred to this primitive mode of perception where any change in the perceptual field causes the whole structure of that field to be altered. Gradually, however, the organism becomes more active and able to integrate the incoming data from the sense organs with previous experience. Perception is thus finally stabilized by our capacity to modify the incoming pattern of stimulation to provide a degree of perceptual constancy. By such processes we reduce, organize, and interpret the otherwise chaotic flow of information reaching consciousness to a limited number of differentiated, stable, and meaningful percepts from which our reality is constructed.

During subsequent development, another important process of selection develops which allows us to master our environment in an economic manner. Activities which are repeated over a period of time tend to become automatic and function spontaneously with the minimal utilization of voluntary attention.

This removal of certain ego functions from conscious attention corresponds of course to the Freudian concept of preconscious function. Kubie (1954) describes this process in the following way:

> Preconscious processes drop out of the central focus of consciousness through repetition. Thus all simple activities of life such as breathing, sucking, excreting, moving, crying, are originally random and often explosive acts. Early in life their purposeful execution is learned through repetition, by which they become economically organized into synergistic, goal-directed patterns. As any such act is fully learned, it can be initiated simply by a contemplation of its goal; and as this happens we gradually become unaware of the intermediate steps which make up the act. This great economy is achieved in the process of learning by repetition. It is in this way that we become able to walk without pondering each step, to talk without working out the movements by which we enunciate each word. . . . The importance of this preconscious system of conscious function cannot be overestimated. . . . It is inconceivable that we could have any scientific, artistic, literary, mathematical, or indeed any creative functions without the capacity for enormous economies which preconscious processes possess.

In his analysis of skilled performance Welford (1958) makes the interesting suggestion that "the decision mechanism" of conscious attention is concerned with "the resolution of uncertainty." He describes this process as follows. "More generally the view seems to be tenable that what we recognize as consciousness in the full sense—as opposed to merely not being asleep—arises essentially when some uncertainty requires to be resolved and that the apparent loss of conscious control in highly practised skills is a result of the virtual elimination of uncertainty in performance. . . . On this view, when a performance is so thoroughly learned that it becomes 'automatic,' it can be carried on while leaving the decision mechanism virtually free." Thus, by repetition and the resolution of uncertainty, conscious attention becomes less bound to concrete stimulation and freer to participate in higher mental processes where uncertainty plays a dominant role.

Although it seems unlikely that we can ever define consciousness in purely physiological terms, work in recent years has certainly provided us with evidence for some neurological correlates of conscious mental activity. The role of the brainstem reticular system now appears to be central to the development of conscious functions and it now seems likely that this system makes possible the selective monitoring of incoming information upon which adequate ego functioning is dependent. Brain (1958) concludes his survey of the reticular system's relationship with the process of attention by declaring ". . . it looks rather as though its (the reticular system) function were to prepare not only the cortex but the other sensory pathways also to respond to a sensory impulse when it has arrived. As we have seen, such responses are at least twofold, namely the reduction of other sensory 'information' which might compete for attention, and the integration of the sensory 'information' being attended to with the continuously changing background of somatic and environmental sensory data." Penfield (1954) in his concept of the centrencephalic system reaches the following somewhat similar conclusion, ". . . the hypothesis is suggested that sensory information is integrated within the centrencephalic system. A selected portion of this information is then somehow projected upwards to the temporal cortex by the portion of the system which is in functional connexion with the temporal cortex of both sides. As it is thus projected, a comparison is made with past similar experiences, thanks to records of the past that are held there, and judgement with regard to familiarity and significance is made." Here, it would seem, is the "spotlight" of attention which allows us to deal with our environment in an economic and effective manner.

Now let us suppose that there is a breakdown in this selective-inhibitory function of attention. Consciousness would be flooded with an undifferentiated mass of incoming sensory data, transmitted from the environment via the sense organs. To this involuntary tide of impressions there would be added the diverse internal images, and their associations, which would no longer be coordinated with incoming information. Perception would revert to the passive and involuntary assimilative process of early childhood and, if the incoming flood were to carry on unchecked, it would gradually sweep away the stable constructs of a former reality. Let us now summarize the findings of the present clinical study with this picture in mind.

The schizophrenic patients in the present study describe, at times vividly, the primitive, global, and undifferentiated nature of their perceptions. Recently a number of investigations have been reported dealing with disturbances of perception in mental illness and there is now sufficient experimental evidence to support the assertion that perceptual constancy and selectivity are disturbed particularly in the case of schizophrenia. Wechowicz (1957) and Wechowicz, Sommer, and Hall (1958) have reported a disturbance in both distance and size constancy in chronic schizophrenic patients. Commenting on their findings they declared that "Schizophrenic patients live in a visual world which is lacking in depth (three dimensionality) and the perception of these patients is more literal and less related to the third dimension than the perception of normals." Our patients' comments indicate the same concrete response to the environment and a disturbed perceptual constancy. Their descriptions also imply some degree of perceptual fusion of normally discrete sensory channels, further evidence of a primitivization of the whole perceptual process.

The loss of spontaneity in behavior which they describe would seem to be a natural consequence of their conscious attention being invaded by the volitional impulses and stimuli from the effectors which normally function autonomously outside of the range of awareness. The patient now has consciously to initiate and control his bodily movements, every one of which involves a decision. Activities which were before self-regulative are now experienced as uncertain and requiring deliberate coordination. It is small wonder that the patient speaks of a split between his mind and body, and feels that he is in danger of losing control over his own actions.

The patient finds difficulty in ordering, not only his movements, but also his thoughts. Like his movements the patient's thoughts are nonvolitional, uncoordinated, and subject to sudden stops. The disturbance of thinking again reflects the fundamental loss of the normal mechanism of selective-inhibitory control of attention. This conclusion is in accordance with the many studies already made of schizophrenic thought disorders which invariably reach one conclusion in common. Schilder (1951) speaks of the schizophreni-patient being ". . . unable to pursue the determinative idea." Cameron (1944) refers to over-inclusion "as a central factor in schizophrenic thought disorder," while Arieti (1955) speaks of ". . . a lack of inhibition of peripheral ideas necessary for effective abstraction." McKellar (1957) explains the loss of abstract thinking in schizophrenia as being due to "the inability to inhibit associated but irrelevant ideas." In a report of a recent investigation carried out at the Maudsley Hospital the main conclusion was as follows: "Overinclusive thinking is due to a defect in some central filter which is responsible for screening out stimuli, both internal and external, which are irrelevant to the task in hand. . . . This filter presumably operates by inhibiting those stimuli by some process similar to that described by Pavlov. . . . It is conceivable that schizophrenics are abnormal in that they do not readily develop any kind of cortical inhibition" (Payne, Mattussek, and George, 1959). In a recent paper (Wechowicz and Blewett, 1959) the relationship between one aspect of perceptual disorder, size constancy and the disturbance of abstract thinking in chronic schizophrenics has been examined, and the findings here tend to confirm a correlation between perceptual constancy and abstract thinking. These authors conclude that the abnormalities of thinking and perception in schizophrenic patients are secondary and causally related to a basic inability to attend selectively to the incoming sensory input from the environment. The clinical findings in the present study would appear to point in the same direction, suggesting that the disturbances of perception and thinking in early schizophrenics are secondary to the primary disturbances in the control of the direction of attention.

We have already considered the affective changes which take place and argued that these are secondary and consequent upon the basic cognitive disturbance. It would seem to us, in fact, that all other apparently irrational features of schizophrenic behaviour also represent attempts made by the patient to cope with, and rationalize, his changing experience. Many of the apparently bizarre and meaningless activities of schizophrenic patients become more rational if we consider their function in aiding the patient to find a new level of adaptation. This goes beyond the scope of the present discussion, but we might cite the example of several patients whose habit of stuffing their ears with cotton wool and closing their eyes becomes more intelligible once the defensive function of their actions was understood. One might also note in passing that if our view of schizophrenic experience is correct then the paranoid patient's description of a hostile environment which seeks to control him is perhaps a valid reflexion of his view of reality.

From the point of view of etiology, it would seem that if schizophrenia is a disease which has its basic effect in a disruption of the control of attention then the reticular system may be the main pathological site.

Symonds (1954), in his discussion of the reticular system, makes the following comments which appear to us to be highly relevant to the present subject:

> There is much evidence suggesting the existence of tonic activity from the cortex, and probably from the brain stem and cerebellum, having an inhibitory effect on synapses of the afferent pathways. . . . Further studies on the unanaesthetized cat by means of implanting electrodes suggests that inhibition of afferent inflow may be selective and its direction governed by attention so that, for example, impulses set up in the visual pathways by photic stimulation are depressed when the animal is at the same time exposed to auditory or olfactory stimulus. . . . If it is accepted that the afferent flow to the cortex is thus subject to voluntary control, what might happen if this control were withdrawn?

Although Symonds was not considering mental illness in his discussion, the answer to his last question concerning a breakdown in the reticular system, resulting in the cortex being bombarded with irrelevant information, might be schizophrenia. It may be pertinent that the tranquilizing drugs which are most effective in schizophrenia are thought to operate by exercising an inhibitory effect upon subcortical areas, including that covered by the reticular system.

## A Proposed Study of Early Schizophrenia

A clinical study of the phenomena reported by early schizophrenics has led us to a hypothesis that might be stated as follows: The earliest reported symptoms of a schizophrenic illness indicate that a primary disorder is that of a decrease in the selective and inhibitory functions of attention. The disturbance in this process leads to a number of other pathological changes which include:

1. A primitivization of the perceptual process resulting in a gradual tendency for perception to become global, undifferentiated, and lacking in spatio-temporal constancy.
2. A progressive diffuseness in the operation of hitherto discrete sensory channels, which may be likened to the phenomenon of synesthesia.
3. Disturbances in the control and direction of motility or willed action which appears as a heightened awareness of bodily functions and volitional impulses which are normally outside of the range of conscious awareness.
4. A decrease in concentration and progressive thought disorder related to the basic inability to abstract from the incoming flow of information and its internal association that which is pertinent to a logical sequence of thinking.

The most obvious way of testing the validity of this hypothesis would take the form of a further, more intensive examination of a group of established schizophrenic patients. There are, however, two main disadvantages to this approach. The initial selection of the subjects is dependent upon the classical diagnosis of schizophrenia which is subject to observer variation. In order to overcome diagnostic difficulties it is thus necessary to confine one's investigation to schizophrenic patients whose symptoms are of long duration, where the course of the disease has placed the diagnosis beyond doubt. This restriction of examination to chronic schizophrenic patients raises the second difficulty, in that evidence of the primary disorder in such patients is apt to be obscured by the secondary reactions and the general deterioration which is consequent upon the chronic state. The methodology of investigation is further limited by the relative inaccessibility of many chronic patients and their inability to act as reliable subjects in experimental procedures. In view of these difficulties it is intended to confine the proposed investigation to patients who are as yet in the early stages of their illness. It is hoped to circumvent some of the uncertainties of early diagnosis by widening the investigation to include all patients presented for their first psychiatric consultation within a stated age range (17–25 years), *regardless* of the psychiatric diagnosis made on referral. Each patient will be observed over a period of time by means of a standardized interview technique and by a series of experimental methods designed to assess the hypothetical phenomena already outlined. According to the findings provided by these two independent sets of data, it should be possible to isolate those patients whose responses show a pattern in accordance with our hypothesis. The remaining patients will of course then automatically function as controls. The patients will be subsequently followed up, their psychiatric progress assessed at a later date and subsequently compared with the clinical and experimental findings.

These experimental techniques have been designed to examine objectively each of the areas of cognitive change reported by the patients in the present clinical study. By these methods it is hoped to obtain indices representing pathological changes in such functions as that of selective attention, perceptual stability, and sequential thinking. Particular attention will be paid to the influence of stimulation in one sensory channel on the output of alternative channels, in an attempt to isolate the phenomenon of perceptual "fusion" which is so characteristic of the reports of schizophrenic patients. Some indication of disorder in the field of motility will be obtained by selected tests of the effect produced by visual and auditory stimulation on motor performance.

This clinical-experimental approach provides a means of testing the hypothesis that certain schizophrenic symptoms are a result of a disturbance in the selective-inhibitory mechanism of attention. The findings of the investigation may also add to our competence in making an early differential diagnosis of schizophrenia. One of the current beliefs in some quarters of psychiatry is that clinical psychiatry need no longer be concerned with the field of psychotic illness, which is proving to be a biochemical problem, the solution to which will some day be provided by the biochemists. While one does not doubt that ultimately the contributions of biochemistry and neurophysiology will play a decisive role in delineating the etiological factors behind the schizophrenic disturbance, there seems little doubt that clinical psychiatry must still be an active participant. Indeed, one might argue that there is little chance of the organic components of the illness being identified until psychiatry can provide a more exacting classification of schizophrenic disorders. To do this we must seek to define and measure schizophrenic states in a more specific and detailed way, keeping in mind the possible organic implications of our clinical findings. If psychiatry can perform this task efficiently it might then be possible to approach the biochemist and neurophysiologist with a set of clearly defined questions to which there would be some possibility of an answer. Schizophrenia, which has so long eluded our full understanding, is much too complex a problem ever to be solved by an approach limited to one method of inquiry. It requires an approach, which in terminology, methodology and theoretical construction, is flexible enough to embrace the whole field of psychiatric research. In the development of our own thinking on this subject we have found it necessary to go a long way from our original psychoanalytic framework and have expanded it to include concepts taken from clinical psychiatry, developmental and experimental psychology, and from neurophysiology. Such an eclectic approach seems to us to be demanded by a subject which lies at the focal point of many disciplines.

Finally, we should like to emphasize the value of careful clinical observation in any study of schizophrenic patients. Although we propose to complement our clinical findings with information obtained by experimental methods, we do not mean to imply that the latter type of data is necessarily more objective and "respectable," or that upon it depends the validity of the clinical material. Clinical observations may provide their own internal criterion of validity, *if* they are made in a controlled and systematic way. We are well aware that the observations upon which the present paper is founded have been collected in a manner which does not comply with these conditions. They have, however, led to the formulation of a hypothesis which can be subjected to a more rigorous evaluation. It is our hope that the reporting of the observations made by these patients will serve to accentuate the primary role which clinical observation must play in the development of any constructive theory of schizophrenia.

## REFERENCES

Arieti, S., *Interpretation of Schizophrenia* (New York: Robert Brunner, 1955).

Brain, R., "The Psychological Basis of Consciousness," *Brain,* 81 (1958), 426.

Cameron, N., "An Experimental Analysis of Schizophrenic Thinking," in J. S. Kasanin, ed., *Language and Thought in Schizophrenia* (Berkeley: University of California Press, 1944).

Chapman, J., T. F. Freeman, and A. McGhie, "Clinical Research in Schizophrenia—The Psychotherapeutic Approach," *Brit. J. Med. Psychol.,* 32 (1959), 2.

Delafresnaye, J. F., ed., *Brain Mechanisms and Consciousness* (Oxford: Blackwell Scientific Publications, 1954).

Federn, P., *Ego Psychology and the Psychoses* (London: Imago Publishing, 1953).

Freeman, T., and A. McGhie, "The Relevance of Genetic Psychology for the Psychopathology of Schizophrenia," *Brit. J. Med. Psychol.,* 30 (1957), 176.

Freeman, T., J. L. Cameron, and A. McGhie, *Chronic Schizophrenia* (London: Tavistock Publications Ltd., 1958).

Jung, R., "Correlations of Bioelectrical and Autonomic Phenomena with Alterations of Consciousness and Arousal in Man," in J. F. Delafresnaye, ed., *Brain Mechanisms and Consciousness* (Oxford: Blackwell Scientific Publications, 1954).

Kubie, L. F., "Psychiatric and Psychoanalytic Considerations of the Problem of Consciousness," in J. F. Delafresnaye, ed., *op. cit.*

Payne, R. W., P. Mattussek, and E. I. George, "An Experimental Study of Schizophrenic Thought Disorder," *J. Ment. Sci.,* 105 (1959), 440.

McKellar, P., *Imagination and Thinking* (London: Cohen and West, 1957).

Penfield, W., "Studies of the Cerebral Cortex in Man—A Review and Interpretation," in J. F. Delafresnaye, ed., *op. cit.*

Piaget, J., *Play, Dreams and Imitation in Childhood* (London: Heinemann, 1951).

Schilder, P., *Brain and Personality* (New York: International Univer-sities Press, 1951).

Symonds, C. P., "Cataplexy and Other Related Forms of Seizure," *Canad. Med. Ass. J.*, 70 (1954), 621.

Wechowicz, T. E., "Size Constancy in Schizophrenic Patients," *J. Ment. Sci.*, 103 (1957), 432.

Wechowicz, T. E., R. Sommer, and R. Hall, "Distance Constancy in Schizophrenic Patients," *J. Ment. Sci.*, 104 (1958), 436.

Wechowicz, T. E., and D. B. Blewett, "Size Constancy and Abstract Thinking in Schizophrenic Patients," *J. Ment. Sci.*, 105 (1959), 441.

Welford, A. T., *Ageing and Human Skill* (New York: Oxford University Press, 1958).

# 3 : A Learning Theory Approach to Research in Schizophrenia

SARNOFF A. MEDNICK

This paper is concerned with some aspects of schizophrenic behavior that seem amenable to interpretation in terms of learning theory. There is no pretense of completeness or uniqueness of explanation, univocal experimental support or lack of other theories to explain the same behavior. The advantage of this explanation has been the readiness with which it is tested, the success of the tests, and the support which the clinical literature lends.

The discussion will take the following form. (*a*) First we will review certain experiments studying the conditioning, generalization, and learning of schizophrenics, and show how these results can be understood in terms of learning theory. (*b*) We will attempt to outline some possible conditions for the onset

Reprinted by permission of the author and publisher from *Psychological Bulletin*, 55 (1958), 316–27. The work reported here was supported by Research Grant M–1519 from the National Institute of Mental Health.

of the thinking disorder in schizophrenia. Here we will be suggesting that generalization and high levels of anxiety may be mutually supportive and augmentative; generalization under these conditions may thus become excessive, leading to difficulties in sequential thought. (*c*) The nature of the explanation of the thinking disorder will suggest the reason for the transition from the acute to the chronic phase of the illness. The thinking of abstracted, irrelevant thoughts may be rewarded by anxiety reduction by removing disturbing ideation from consciousness. This would increase the probability of the recurrence of these irrelevant thoughts and would be an admirable vehicle for continual anxiety reduction and transition to a chronic phase.

## Research on Conditioning, Learning, and Generalization

The lack of anxiety of the schizophrenic, often considered an aspect of "flat affect" or emotionlessness, has received considerable attention in the clinical and experimental literature.[1,4,6,30] This reduction in reactivity has also been the focus of many theoretical discussions of the disorder. However, while "flat affect" might be a term descriptive of certain schizophrenic patients (mainly chronic, although even this has been questioned[41]), it has not normally been used in describing the incipient or acute patient. Thus, Arieti calls the first stage of schizophrenia "a period of intense anxiety and panic." Experimental studies seem to suggest that the acute patient is very reactive, showing extreme anxiety.[13,36,39,61,74,79] Research also suggests that such an emotionally disturbed individual will take longer to recover from an affective imbalance than will normals.[13, 14, 79] This hyperreactivity has manifested itself in studies of heart rate, the psychogalvanic response, startle reflex, reactions to painful stimulations, and so on. These studies seem to point to a low threshold of emotional arousal in at least the acute schizophrenic. Recent work in the area of conditioning and learning has identified states of emotional arousal as contributing (as do states such as hunger and thirst) to drive strength, a construct postulated by Hull to represent the motivational force of the behavior of the organism.[19]

All of the above may be taken to suggest that acute schizophrenics are organisms in a state of heightened drive. Hull's theory[29] and extensions of this theory make specific predictions of the effect of this heightened drive state on behavior. In general, the effect of heightened drive is to increase the response strength of any habit tendencies that may be aroused in a given situation. Thus, in general, the hungrier, or more anxious, or more fearful the organism, the greater his drive and the greater the speed and amplitude of his responses.

In a simple conditioning situation where the number of response alternatives is restricted (usually to one possible response) high drive would augment the response strength of the conditioned response. Thus, a group with high drive (in this case schizophrenics) should show faster conditioning than a low drive group. There have been some studies that indicate that schizophrenics can be conditioned.[5, 25, 37, 51, 59] Other studies have compared schizophrenics with control groups for ease of conditioning. The earliest of these is the study by Pfaffman and Schlosberg.[58] They conditioned the knee-jerk response in 25 schizophrenics and 25 normal Ss. The schizophrenics conditioned faster. A study by Mays[42] and a study by Shipley[70] indicate that schizophrenics show faster conditioning of the psychogalvanic response than do normals. Recent studies by Taylor and Spence, and Spence and Taylor, indicate that schizophrenics show faster eye blink conditioning than normals or anxiety neurotics[73,76]. The results of these several studies support the above prediction that schizophrenics show faster conditioning than normals.

*Stimulus generalization.* When a response, having been trained to a stimulus, is also elicited by similar stimuli, stimulus generalization may be said to have occurred. As pointed out above, the effect of increased drive is to increase the response strength of aroused habit tendencies. As a consequence, high drive tends to produce heightened generalization responsiveness. It is, therefore, reasonable to expect, on the basis of these speculations, that schizophrenics would show elevated generalization responsivity.

On the basis of clinical observation, Schilder[67] first remarked on the difficulties schizophrenics have in tasks involving differentiation. Bender and Schilder, studying conditioned withdrawal from shock,[5] noted extreme overgeneralization from their schizophrenic *S*s. Cameron has spoken of overinclusion and the broadening of the generalization gradient on the part of schizophrenics.[7, 8, 10] Garmezy,[21] studying generalization along the dimension of pitch, found schizophrenics showing more generalization than normals. This effect was especially marked under conditions of stress (strong drive arousal). Mednick, using the dimension of space, found that schizophrenics, especially acute patients, generalized more than normals.[44, 45] Dunn tested schizophrenics with social and nonsocial materials, finding, with social materials, greater generalization than was shown by the control group.[17]

The several studies cited support the prediction that schizophrenics show elevated generalization responsivity.

*Complex learning.* For purposes of this discussion a complex learning task will be defined as a situation in which many irrelevant and incorrect habit tendencies are aroused with which the correct response must compete. For example, in the serial learning of a word list, words other than the next correct response are potential competing responses. In this context high drive, acting impartially upon correct and incorrect response tendencies, will tend to push many irrelevant responses above the evocation threshold.[20, 75] The suprathreshold irrelevant tendencies will interfere with the correct responses, causing a relatively large number of errors and relatively slow attainment of a list criterion. Thus, in contrast to the conditioning-type situation, it is predicted that in complex response situations schizophrenics will reach a criterion more slowly than normals and with more errors. Relative to this prediction there is a considerable array of studies demonstrating poor performance by schizophrenics in complex tasks.[4, 30, 31] The Es often report that the schizophrenics' performance is retarded by irrelevant, incorrect responses. For example, Cameron's concept of interpenetration might be understood in these terms.[9] A paired-associate verbal learning study by Hall and Crookes showed schizophrenics performing less well than normals. Hall and Crookes attribute the poor performance to extralist intrusion.[26] As pointed out above, Hullian theory would explain this in terms of high drive indiscriminately increasing the probability of remote, irrelevant responses being evoked.

As defined above, a paired-associate verbal learning task is a very complex task. However, the complexity can be minimized in several ways. Intralist similarity and intralist cross associates could be largely eliminated. Words which are already dominant associates can be chosen as the response members of the associate pairs; this would make the most probable associates correct and eliminate them as possible interfering tendencies. Such a list of paired associates would contain pairs such as "black-white" and "table-chair." While this list minimizes the possibility of competing responses, such responses are still very possible. However, in this relatively low complexity situation the present orientation would predict that the schizophrenics would learn the list at *least* as quickly as normals and with *at least* a comparable number of errors. The "at least" refers to the possibility that complexity is so reduced that the task approaches the level of a conditioning situation. If the task is of low enough complexity the schizophrenic should then perform better than the normals.

The complexity of a paired-associate list may also be maximized. An example of such a list may be illustrated by the associate pairs:

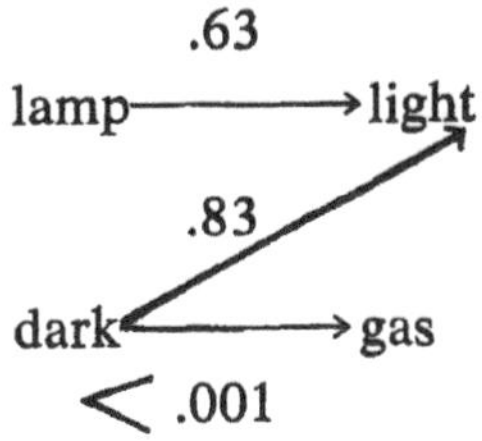


While in the low complexity list we took the most probable word associate to a stimulus word and made it the correct response, in this maximum competition list we have made it an incorrect response. As noted, the probability of associating "gas" to "dark" is less than one in a thousand,[65] while the probability of associating "light" to "dark" is .83. Thus, "light" is a highly probable erroneous response to the stimulus "dark." In view of the low probability of the "dark-gas" pair other erroneous associates to "dark" such as "night" also have a high probability of evocation. High drive will tend to arouse relatively more erroneous associates and will give these associates relatively greater response strength. Thus schizophrenics would be predicted to make more errors and to take longer to learn a high complexity list. Mednick and DeVito[48] compared the learning of schizophrenics and normals on such minimum and maximum complexity lists. The schizophrenic Ss learned the low complexity list more quickly than the normals, while the normals learned the high complexity list more quickly. The interaction of Groups X Lists was very highly significant ($F = 258.1$ at 1, 82 *df*).

Another instance of the increasing difficulty schizophrenics have as a function of increasing task complexity is described by Hunt and Cofer. From the rich data collected by the Worcester State Hospital group[32] in the 1930's, Hunt and Cofer compared the difference in the performance of normals and schizophrenics in reflex time, simple reaction time, and discrimination reaction time, tasks which are graded in complexity. Hunt and Cofer comment from an analysis of this and other data ". . . we have quantitative evidence that the deficit becomes greater as the complexity of the task increases."[31]

Thus, three characteristics of schizophrenic behavior which reliably distinguish them from normals are: (*a*) schizophrenics more easily acquire a conditioned response; (*b*) schizophrenics show greater stimulus generalization responsiveness; (*c*) schizophrenics have great difficulty performing well in complex situations, being plagued by irrelevant, tangential associative responses competing with the adequate mode of response. However, they do *at least* as well as normals on low complexity tasks.

In the framework of the present orientation all of these behavioral characteristics would be predicted in a group with extremely high drive.

### *The Thinking Disorder*

Bleuler considered the "disturbances of association" a primary symptom of schizophrenia from which the other disordered behaviors stem.

> It appears as if those pathways of association and inhibition established by experience had lost their meaning and significance. Associations seem to take new pathways more easily, and thus no longer follow the old preferred ways, that is, the logical pathways indicated by past experience. . . . Especially in acute conditions of schizophrenia, one often finds so complete a fragmentation of the thinking processes that they cannot result in a complete idea or action.[6]

Cameron and Magaret described the disorder of thinking in much the same way.

> Contradictory, competing, and more or less irrelevant responses can no longer be excluded. . . . Schizophrenic patients themselves often complain about the confusion in their talk and thinking, saying that everything seems mixed up, the words do not come as they once did, thoughts rush in and are jumbled. . . . "There are a million words," one patient said, "I can't make sentences; everything is disconnected." Another patient made several attempts to speak and then gave up; the next day

she complained her thoughts had been rushing through her mind so that she could say nothing.[11]

Observers differ in their theoretical interpretation of the thinking disorder. Cameron refers to desocialization.[11] Kraepelin speaks of disconnection of thought;[34] Goldstein[22] interprets the disorder in terms of an impairment of abstract behavior; habit deterioration is Meyer's explanation;[49] Pavlov[57] understands it as a sensitization caused by overstimulation leading to a condition of cortical inhibition; Hanfmann and Kasanin refer to a loss of generalizing ability.[27] Bateson uses the concept of the double bind;[2] Shakow notes the importance of the inability to maintain a set.[69]

While these workers may differ in their theory, they will probably acknowledge that the statements of Bleuler and Cameron and Magaret describe the behavior they seek to explain. This thought disorganization resulting from "irrelevant," "fragmented," and "competing" associations may also be understood in terms of the framework here presented. In terms of the above definition, thinking is perhaps the most complex behavior in which man can engage. There are thousands of verbal thought units that potentially compete with the single thought unit that may be demanded by a given context. (For purposes of this discussion a verbal thought unit may be informally defined as a major form class, a verb, an adjective, or noun.) These competitors may be synonyms, symbolic representatives, word associates, clang associates, and so on.[12, 15, 35, 43, 54, 60, 66] Due to previous association, or similarity of meaning or sound, some thought units are probable or strong competitors. Others, more remote and irrelevant, rarely have enough response strength to reach awareness. Predictions from an extension of Hullian theory would suggest that the thinking of individuals with high drive would be disrupted by the intrusion of the remote and irrelevant thought units pushed above the threshold of awareness. The writer suggests that this action of high drive upon remote response tendencies is a major root of the disordered thinking of schizophrenics. In support of this hypothesis, a recent study by M. Mednick shows that relatively remote associations have more response strength for high anxious than for low anxious normals.[43]

It may be instructive to make use of this general framework to attempt to briefly explain the possible origins of what Arieti calls the first stage of schizophrenia where the thinking disorder originally manifests itself. This description of the development of the schizophrenic break grew from attempts at explaining the conditions for the onset of illness as it was described by early acute schizophrenics. It tries to reflect their feeling of being caught in expanding, spiralling vortexes of anxiety and ideation, reciprocally supporting and augmenting each other. It also tries to remember that many of these early schizophrenics will go on to become chronic. Unless the acute and chronic phases are two separate illnesses, it seems likely that a *single set of principles should explain both states.*

To begin with, the preschizophrenic is an extremely anxious individual.[1, 39, 40] (The possible explanations for this may run the gamut from endocrinological to psyschoanalytic to learning theories but will not be the concern of this paper.) In other words, he is an individual who strongly fears many stimulus situations. His high drive level causes him to display an abnormal amount of stimulus and associative generalization.[3, 43, 46, 63, 64, 78] This means that stimulus events that are in some way similar to the stimulus situations he has learned to fear will also tend to elicit anxiety responses. (These stimulus events include thoughts.)

Some cases learn to restrict their contact with anxiety provoking events and thoughts inasmuch as this avoidance is reinforced by anxiety reduction.[50] Since they avoid potential anxiety-producing situations, learned anxiety never extinguishes.[72] In most cases, this borderline adjustment continues through life and is usually termed withdrawn or schizoid.

In many cases, however, some life crisis or an untoward incident (later called the "precipitating event") interferes with this adjustment. This crisis or incident may take the form of the termination of adolescence, homosexual panic, an auto accident, the death of a loved one, or simply some morbid ruminating. In any case, the event is one which will raise the individual's anxiety level. For the highly anxious preschizophrenic, this imbalance is a serious affair which may have alarming ramifications. For one thing, the high-anxious person will have a relatively large anxiety response to the precipitating incident. This will temporarily push his total drive state up to unusually high levels. One important consequence of this will be the attendant increase in the level and breadth of generalization responsivity. While he previously reacted with fear to many stimulus situations, the increase in generalization will cause a large number of new stimuli to become potential anxiety arousers. The high-anxious individual finds that some of the stimuli which were once safe and comfortable for him now fill him with uneasiness. While he once felt comfortable in the presence of his superior, the incremented gradient of fear stemming from learned reactions to his father now cause him to experience discomfort.

Not only does the increase in generalization increase the number of stimuli which will arouse a fear response, it also augments the amplitude of response to the old fear producing stimuli. The low-anxious individual can usually allow his anxiety level to "simmer down" by means of a good night's sleep. The high-anxious person will find it hard to sleep; the pressure of the greatly increased anxiety keeps thoughts running through his mind. The thoughts will be partially cued by the ongoing anxiety state and may relate to other periods of disturbance, causing still more upset.

In summary, we find that this precipitating incident has a number of uncomfortable consequences. The consequences enumerated above will tend to increase the individual's anxiety level. Unfortunately, this will, in turn, serve to again raise the level and breadth of generalization responsiveness. Again, the effect of this will be to increase the probability of his encountering a fear-arousing stimulus by increasing the number of such stimuli. Also, the amount of fear that a previously adequate stimulus could arouse will be increased. Again, the individual's total anxiety level is likely to continue to rise. Subjectively, the individual will begin to feel very uncomfortable. Things which he could depend on to keep his anxiety down don't work any more. The afternoon beer does not calm anymore; the bartender now makes him feel a bit uneasy. Also, situations which made him bearably anxious now tax his ability to control himself.

Assuming continued stimulation from the world and/or continued thinking, this reciprocal augmentation of anxiety and generalization could theoretically continue unabated until some upper physiological limit of anxiety and/or generalization is reached. Long before this point is reached, however, the behavior of the individual will become noticeably unusual. His drive level will keep thoughts racing through his mind. Many of these thoughts will be out of context or silly. His fear regarding the "craziness" and uncontrolled nature of his thoughts only serves to increase the insistence of these thoughts. The sudden lack of control he has over these thoughts will seem inexplicable. He is either "going crazy" or there is some "rational" solution for all of this. In some cases, because of past experience, a rational solution suggests itself which is compounded of elements such as X-radiation, gamma rays, radio transmitters, and the FBI. This rational solution reduces anxiety more than the thought that he is going crazy. The solution is thus reinforced, increasing the probability of its being called upon as a defense (anxiety reducer) in the presence of inexplicable anxiety or thoughts.

Meanwhile, what is happening to his thinking behavior? As the spiral of anxiety and generalization mounts, his drive level may increase to an almost insupportable degree. As this is taking place, his ability to discriminate is almost totally eclipsed by his generalization tendencies.[67] Any unit of a thought sequence might call up some remote associate and this associate will call up still another remote associate. Clang associates based on stimulus-response generalization may be frequent. Body positions accidentally associated with any fleeting periods of anxiety reduction will tend to be continually and in some cases continuously assumed. These will be rationalized ("If I move, evil will envelop the world.") and may be maintained for long periods of time. His speech may resemble a "word salad." He will be an acute schizophrenic with a full-blown thinking disorder.

Much of the above description of this acute process rests upon the hypothesis of the reciprocal augmentation of anxiety and generalized fear responses. There is some support for an obvious deduction from this hypothesis. The reciprocal augmentation model would predict slower extinction of a learned fear response with massed trials; the longer the time between trials, the greater the opportunity for the fear response from the last trial to decay and drop the total anxiety level back to the resting state. If the trials follow each other rapidly enough, Trial 2 will come at a time when the anxiety from Trial 1 has not yet been dissipated. Thus the total drive state at Trial 2 will be the resting level plus the remaining anxiety from Trial 1. Since the total drive level will be higher on Trial 2 than it was on Trial 1, the stimulus on Trial 2 should elicit an augmented anxiety response. This Trial 2 anxiety response should take longer to decay than that of previous trials and should in the manner outlined lead to an augmented Trial 3 anxiety response, and so on. Response fatigue might dampen this spiral effect somewhat. However, studies by Howat,[28] Mednick,[47] and Murphy and Miller,[53] all using noxious UCS's, have obtained little or no extinction under the conditions of massed trials and relatively rapid extinction under spaced practice.

This explication of the reciprocal augmentation process clarifies an important question. Why doesn't everybody proceed to schizophrenia after an extremely anxiety provoking event?

The answer lies in three factors: the individual's original drive level, his rate of recovery from anxiety states, and the number of stimuli that elicit anxiety responses from the individual.

Highly anxious individuals will tend to have relatively strong anxiety responses. The resultant large increments in drive will take long periods to decay;[14, 16] during these periods drive will continue to remain in a heightened state, leaving the individual prone to be swept up in the reciprocal augmentation spiral.

If an individual has an abnormally slow recovery rate from anxiety arousal, a relatively small arousal state may have a long term effect, equivalent to that of a major anxiety response in a normal individual. During this extended arousal period, responsivity (including anxiety responses) will be heightened and generalization will be increased. Darrow and Heath,[14] Wulfeck,[79] and Cohen and Patterson[13] have demonstrated that schizophrenics and highly anxious persons tend to have an abnormally slow recovery rate from anxiety arousal. This relationship holds even with allowance made for the magnitude of the anxiety response.

Almost by definition, the number of stimuli which elicit anxiety will be higher for the high-anxious person. Thus, he will find it relatively difficult to seek out soothing stimulation or thoughts to help mitigate his response to a crisis. Almost any place he turns will be fraught with aspects that arouse uneasiness. Many thoughts will contain elements which will generalize to anxiety provoking ideas.

Thus, the low-anxious person is not likely to demonstrate a large anxiety response to fear provoking stimuli; his anxiety response will decay relatively rapidly; he will find it relatively easy to avoid further anxiety stimulation. Thus, he is not likely to get enmeshed in the anxiety-generalization spiral unless the precipitating trauma is extremely fear provoking and this type of stimulation continues unabated. Behavior under conditions such as this was studied by Grinker and Spiegel,[23, 24] who observed schizophrenic behavior in otherwise sound individuals who were subjected to the continuous strain of combat in World War II.

It should be clear by now that high drive, slow recovery rate, and number of fear-arousing stimuli are highly correlated factors. A large-anxiety response will take longer to decay. People who give large-anxiety responses will tend to have slower recovery rates. Under conditions of high drive, generalization will be increased making for more stimuli which will elicit anxiety. This, in turn, will produce more anxiety. However, the highly anxious individual may escape the anxiety-generalization spiral by avoiding continued stimulation or by subduing his anxiety level by means of appropriate drugs.[33, 52, 55, 56, 62, 68, 71, 77] This "treatment" will not cure the individual; nor will it prevent breakdown at some later date. However, it may prevent an acute break and lessen the danger that the condition will proceed to chronicity. The source of the anxiety and slow recovery rate must still be ascertained and, if possible, removed before any lasting cure may be said to have been effected. An interesting consideration of some neurophysiological approaches to ascertaining the source of the anxiety arousal is discussed by Malmo.[18, 38]

## The Transition from the Acute to the Chronic Phase

The spiralling process described above has its own built-in stabilizer which leads the patient to chronicity. The stabilizing process is conceived of as follows.

In the midst of this high anxiety state, each time the individual responds with an anxiety-provoking thought the increment in drive will produce an increment in generalization. This may result in a highly generalized, remote, irrelevant, tangential associate. A necessary result of responding with this remote associate is the removal of the anxiety-provoking thought from awareness. Thus, the remote associate will be accompanied by drive reduction, which will reinforce it as a response. This will increase its probability of occurring again in the context of the antecedent anxiety provoking thought or similar thoughts. This process occurring over and over again in many contexts will provide the patient with a repertoire of anxiety-reducing though inappropriate thought response. At first his repertoire may be limited, making for an impression of stereotypy. However, eventually (perhaps after several acute breaks), his thinking will present a varied though disorganized picture. At this point, if the patient, perceiving the disorganization, responds with the anxiety-provoking thought, "I am going crazy," he can defend against it by making an immediate associative transition to an irrelevant, tangential thought or by making use of a well-learned rationale such as "the radiators are broadcasting to me." This disorganized thinking will be continually self-reinforcing since it will enable him to evade anxiety-provoking stimuli. Eventually it will be extremely difficult to reach his awareness for any prolonged period with material that is anxiety provoking. Since he is not dependent on the world for much of his drive reduction, he will become more and more "estranged" from it. What is especially invidious is that he will find these newly-learned techniques extremely effective and efficient in controlling anxiety. The individual need not seek special kinds of stimulation; he need not engage in elaborate rituals; he need not obtain special equipment. He simply thinks irrelevant thoughts. As the term of his illness increases and he uses these techniques more and more he will demonstrate less and less emotionality. As the patient moves into the chronic phase of the illness he may develop the "flat affect" syndrome. In some cases, the remote associations may impel to action. In others, certain actions or postures may have regularly accompanied early conditions of drive reduction and may have been incidentally learned. These postures or mannerisms will tend to be repeated and to be called on to reduce anxiety.

It may be important to note that even the chronic patient is in one sense a very anxious person. He has never had the opportunity to extinguish his prepsychotic fears. They are still elicitable; all that is required is that one break through the schizophrenic's "associative curtain."

## SUMMARY

An attempt has been made to view schizophrenia as a problem in learning theory. The research in conditioning, learning, and generalization in schizophrenia has been reviewed in these terms. It was found that this research supported such an interpretation.

An explication of the causes of an acute schizophrenic break and the transition to chronicity was attempted.

## REFERENCES

1. Arieti, S., *Interpretation of Schizophrenia* (New York: Robert Brunner, 1955).
2. Bateson, G., D. D. Jackson, J. Haley, and J. Weakland, "Toward a Theory of Schizophrenia," *Behav. Sci.*, 1 (1956), 251–64.
3. Beach, F. A., "Effects of Testosterone Propionate on Copulatory Behavior of Sexually Inexperienced Male Rats," *J. Comp. Psychol.*, 33 (1942), 227–47.
4. Bellak, L., and Elizabeth Wilson, "On the Etiology of Dementia Praecox; A Partial Review of the Literature 1935–1945 and an Attempt at Conceptualization," *J. Nerv. Ment. Dis.*, 105 (1947), 1–24.
5. Bender, L., and P. Schilder, "Unconditioned Reactions to Pain in Schizophrenia," *Amer. J. Psychiat.*, 10 (1930), 365–84.
6. Bleuler, E., *Dementia Praecox or the Group of Schizophrenias* (New York: International Universities Press, 1950), pp. 349–50.
7. Cameron, N., "Reasoning, Regression and Communication in Schizophrenics," *Psychol. Monogr.*, 50 (1938), No. 1 (whole No. 221).
8. Cameron, N., "Schizophrenic Thinking in a Problem-Solving Situation," *J. Ment. Sci.*, 85 (1939), 1–24.
9. Cameron, N., "The Functional Psychoses," in J. McV. Hunt, ed., *Personality and the Behavior Disorders* (2 vols., New York: Ronald, 1944).

10. Cameron, N., "Perceptual Organization and Behavior Pathology," in R. R. Blake and G. V. Ramsey, eds., *Perception, an Approach to Personality* (New York: Ronald, 1951).
11. Cameron, N., and A. Magaret, *Behavior Pathology* (Boston: Houghton Mifflin, 1951), p. 511.
12. Cofer, C. N., and J. P. Foley, Jr., "Mediated Generalization and the Interpretation of Verbal Behavior: I. Prolegomena," *Psychol. Rev.*, 49 (1942), 513–40.
13. Cohen, L. H., and M. Patterson, "Effect of Pain on the Heart Rate of Normal and Schizophrenic Individuals," *J. Gen. Psychol.*, 17 (1937), 273–79.
14. Darrow, C. W., and L. L. Heath, "Reaction Tendencies Related to Personality," in K. S. Lashley, ed., *Studies in the Dynamics of Behavior* (Chicago: University of Chicago Press, 1932).
15. Diven, K. E., "Certain Determinants in the Conditioning of Anxiety Reactions," *J. Psychol.*, 3 (1937), 291–308.
16. Duffy, E., "The Psychological Significance of the Concept of 'Arousal' or 'Activation,'" *Psychol. Rev.*, 64 (1957), 265–75.
17. Dunn, W. L., "Visual Discrimination of Schizophrenic Subjects as a Function of Stimulus Meaning," *J. Pers.*, 23 (1954), 48–64.
18. Eccles, J. C., *The Neurophysiological Basis of Mind* (Oxford: Clarendon, 1953).
19. Farber, I. E., "Anxiety as a Drive State," in M. R. Jones, ed., *Nebraska Symposium on Motivation* (Lincoln: Nebraska University Press, 1954).
20. Farber, I. E., and K. W. Spence, "Complex Learning and Conditioning as a Function of Anxiety," *J. Exp. Psychol.*, 45 (1953), 120–25.
21. Garmezy, N., "Stimulus Differentiation by Schizophrenic and Normal Ss under Conditions of Reward and Punishment," *J. Pers.*, 20 (1952), 253–76.
22. Goldstein, K., "The Significance of Special Mental Tests for Diagnosis and Prognosis in Schizophrenia," *Amer. J. Psychiat.*, 96 (1939), 575–88.
23. Grinker, R. R., and J. P. Spiegel, *Men Under Stress* (New York: Blakiston, 1945).
24. Grinker, R. R., and J. P. Spiegel, *War Neurosis* (New York: Blakiston, 1945).
25. Guk, E. D., "The Conditioned Reflex Activity of Schizophrenics," *Sovetak. Nevropatol.*, No. 1 (1934), 78–84; English abstract in *Psychological Abstracts*, 9 (1934), 717.
26. Hall, K. R. L., and T. G. Crookes, "Studies in Learning Impairment, I: Schizophrenic and Organic Patients," *J. Ment. Sci.*, 97 (1951), 725–37.
27. Hanfmann, E., and J. Kasanin, "Conceptual Thinking in Schizophrenia," *Nerv. Ment. Dis. Monogr.*, no. 67 (1942).
28. Howat, G., "Influence of Inter-trial Interval during Extinction on 20-minute Spontaneous Recovery of the Conditioned Eyelid Response" (paper presented at Midwest Psychological Association, Chicago, 1957).
29. Hull, C. L., *Principles of Behavior* (New York: Appleton-Century-Crofts, 1943).

30. Hunt, J. McV., "Psychological Experiments with Disordered Persons," *Psychol. Bull.*, 33 (1936), 1–58.
31. Hunt, J. McV., and C. N. Cofer, "Psychological Deficit," in J. McV. Hunt, ed., *Personality and the Behavior Disorders* (New York: Ronald, 1944).
32. Huston, P. E., and D. Shakow, "Learning Capacity in Schizophrenia," *Amer. J. Psychiat.*, 105 (1949), 881–87.
33. Kline, N., and A. M. Stanley, "Use of Reserpine in a Neuropsychiatric Hospital," *Ann. N.Y. Acad. Sci.*, 61 (1955), 85–91.
34. Kraepelin, E., *Clinical Psychiatry* (New York: William Wood, 1917).
35. Lacey, J. I., R. L. Smith, and B. A. Green, "Use of Conditioned Autonomic Responses in the Study of Anxiety," *Psychosom. Med.*, 17 (1955), 208–17.
36. Landis, C., W. A. Hunt, and J. D. Page, "Studies of the Startle Pattern VII. Abnormals," *J. Psychol.*, 4 (1937), 199–206.
37. Landkof, B. L., "Bezuslovnye i Uslovnye Susudistye Reflexi u Schizofrenikov [Unconditioned and Conditioned Vascular Reflexes in Schizophrenia]," *Trud Tsentral Psi Khoevrol Lust.*, 10 (1938), 37–62.
38. Malmo, R. B., "Anxiety and Behavioral Arousal," *Psychol. Rev.*, 64 (1957), 276–87.
39. Malmo, R. B., and C. Shagass, "Physiologic Studies of Reaction to Stress in Anxiety and Early Schizophrenia," *Psychosom. Med.*, 11 (1949), 9–24.
40. Malmo, R. B., C. Shagass, D. J. Belanger, and A. A. Smith, "Motor Control in Psychiatric Patients Under Experimental Stress," *J. Abnorm. Soc. Psychol.*, 46 (1951), 539–47.
41. Malmo, R. B., C. Shagass, and A. A. Smith, "Responsiveness in Chronic Schizophrenia," *J. Pers.*, 4 (1951), 359–75.
42. Mays, L. L., "Studies of Catatonia, V; Investigation of the Perseverational Tendency," *Psychiat. Quart.*, 8 (1934), 728.
43. Mednick, Martha, "Mediated Generalization and the Incubation Effect as a Function of Manifest Anxiety," *J. Abnorm. Soc. Psychol.*, 55 (1957), 315–21.
44. Mednick, S. A., "Distortions of the Gradient of Stimulus Generalization Related to Cortical Brain Damage and Schizophrenia" (doctoral dissertation; Evanston: Northwestern University, 1955).
45. Mednick, S. A., "Distortions in the Gradient of Stimulus Generalization Related to Cortical Brain Damage and Schizophrenia," *J. Abnorm. Soc. Psychol.*, 51 (1955), 536–42.
46. Mednick, S. A., "Generalization as a Function of Manifest Anxiety and Adaptation to Psychological Experiments," *J. Cons. Psych.*, 21 (1957), 491–94.
47. Mednick, S. A., Elizabeth Cope, and Cynthia Wild, "Reciprocal Augmentation of Anxiety and Stimulus Generalization" (unpublished manuscript; Berkeley: Biology Library, University of California).
48. Mednick, S. A., and R. DeVito, "Associative Competition and Verbal Learning in Schizophrenia" (paper read at Eastern Psychological Association, Philadelphia, April 1958).

49. Meyer, A., "Fundamental Conceptions of Dementia Praecox," *J. Nerv. Ment. Dis.*, 34 (1906), 331–36.
50. Miller, N., "Learnable Drives and Rewards," in S. S. Stevens, ed., *Handbook of Experimental Psychology* (New York: John Wiley, 1951).
51. Mirolyubov, N. G., and N. B. Ugol, "The Problem of the State of the Process of Excitation in Schizophrenics," *Sovetsk. Psi. Khenevrol.*, 3 (1933), 68–82; English abstract in *Psychological Abstracts*, 9: 1260 (1935).
52. Monroe, R. R., R. G. Heath, W. A. Mickle, and W. A. Miller, "A Comparison of Cortical and Subcortical Brain Waves in Normal, Barbiturate, Reserpine and Chloropromazine Sleep," *Ann. N.Y. Acad. Sci.*, 61 (1955), 56–71.
53. Murphy, J. V., and R. E. Miller, "Spaced and Massed Practice with a Methodological Consideration of Avoidance Conditioning," *J. Exp. Psychol.*, 52 (1956), 77–81.
54. Noble, C. E., "Conditioned Generalization of the GSR to a Subvocal Stimulus," *J. Exp. Psychol.*, 40 (1950), 15–25.
55. Noce, R. H., D. B. Williams, and W. Rapaport, "Reserpine (Serpasil) in the Management of the Mentally Ill and Mentally Retarded," *J. Amer. Med. Ass.*, 156 (1954), 821–24.
56. Owens, J. W. M., and R. D. Walk, "The Effect of Reserpine on Avoidance Learning" (paper read at Eastern Psychological Association, Atlantic City, April 1956).
57. Pavlov, I. P., *Conditioned Reflexes* (Oxford: Oxford University Press, 1927).
58. Pfaffman, C., and H. Schlosberg, "The Conditioned Knee Jerk in Psychotic and Normal Individuals," *J. Psychol.*, 1 (1935), 201–206.
59. Razran, G., "Withdrawal Responses with Shock as the Conditioning Stimulus in Adult Human Ss," *Psychol. Bull.*, 31 (1934), 111–43.
60. Razran, G., "Semantic and Phonetographic Generalization of Salivary Conditioning to Verbal Stimuli," *J. Exp. Psychol.*, 39 (1949), 642–52.
61. Richter, C. P., "Electrical Skin Resistance, Diurnal and Daily Variation in Psychopathic and Normal Persons," *Arch. Neurol. Psychiat.*, 19 (1928), 488–508.
62. Rinaldi, F., and H. W. Himwich, "A Comparison of the Effects of Reserpine and Some Barbiturates on the Electrical Activity of Cortical and Subcortical Structures of the Brain of Rabbits," *Ann. N.Y. Acad. Sci.*, 61 (1955), 27–35.
63. Rosenbaum, G., "Stimulus Generalization as a Function of Level of Experimentally Produced Anxiety," *J. Exp. Psychol.*, 45 (1953), 35–43.
64. Rosenbaum, G., "Temporal Gradient of Response Strength with Two Levels of Motivation," *J. Exp. Psychol.*, 41 (1951), 261–67.
65. Russell, W. A., and J. J. Jenkins, "The Complete Minnesota Norms for Responses to 100 Words from the Kent-Rosanoff Word Association Test," Technical Report No. 11, ONR Contract N.8, 66216 (Minneapolis: University of Minnesota, 1954).
66. Russell, W. A., and L. H. Storms, "Implicit Verbal Chaining in Paired Associate Learning," *J. Exp. Psychol.*, 49 (1955), 287–93.

67. Schilder, P., "The Psychology of Schizophrenia," *Psychoanal. Rev.*, 26 (1939), 380–98.
68. Schneider, J. A., and A. W. Earl, "Effects of Serpasil on Behavior and Autonomic Regulating Mechanisms," *Neurol.*, 4 (1954), 657–67.
69. Shakow, D., "The Nature of Deterioration in Schizophrenic Conditions," *Nerv. Ment. Dis. Monogr.*, No. 70 (1946).
70. Shipley, W. C., "Studies of Catatonia, VI: Further Investigation of the Perseverative Tendency," *Psychiat. Quart.*, 8 (1934), 736–44.
71. Smith, R. P., A. Wagman, and A. J. Riopelle, "Effects of Reserpine on Conditioned Avoidance Behavior in Normal and Brain-operated Monkeys," *J. Pharm. Exp. Therapeut.*, 117 (1956), 136–41.
72. Solomon, R. L., and E. S. Brush, "Experimentally Derived Conceptions of Anxiety and Aversion," in M. R. Jones, ed., *Nebraska Symposium on Motivation* (Lincoln: University of Nebraska Press, 1956).
73. Spence, K. W., and Janet A. Taylor, "The Relation of CR Strength to Anxiety in Normal, Neurotic, and Psychotic Ss," *J. Exp. Psychol.*, 45 (1953), 265–72.
74. Syz, H. C., "Psychogalvanic Studies in Schizophrenia," *Arch. Neur. Psychiat.*, 16 (1926), 747–60.
75. Taylor, Janet A., "Drive Theory and Manifest Anxiety," *Psychol. Bull.*, 53 (1956), 303–21.
76. Taylor, Janet A., and K. W. Spence," Conditioning Level in the Behavior Disorders," *J. Abnorm. Soc. Psychol.*, 49 (1954), 497–502.
77. Weiskrantz, L., and W. A. Wilson, Jr., "The Effects of Reserpine on Emotional Behavior of Normal and Brain Operated Monkeys," *Ann. N.Y. Acad. Sci.*, 61 (1955), 36–55.
78. Wenar, C., "Reaction Time as a Function of Manifest Anxiety and Stimulus Intensity," *J. Abnorm. Soc. Psychol.*, 48 (1953), 129–34.
79. Wulfeck, W. H., "Motor Function in the Mentally Disordered, I and II," *Psychol. Rec.*, 4 (1941), 271–348.

# 4 : *The Process-Reactive Continuum: A Theoretical Proposal*

ROBERT E. KANTOR

C. L. WINDER

A central psychological postulation is involved in the present proposal: that there are sequential steps of growth which most members of our culture encounter; and that each step contains a central problem which must be at least partially coped with successfully before a new organization of experience can occur adequately on the developmental continuum. To deal successfully with the central problem in any given growth step is what Sullivan called an "integration."

If each core problem is coped with successfully as development proceeds, then regression becomes a very unlikely possibility. In effect, the theory of schizophrenia held in this paper declares that incomplete integrations are antecedents of re-

Reprinted by permission of the authors and publisher from *Journal of Nervous and Mental Disease,* 129 (1959), 429–34.  The paper as it appeared in that journal was a revision of a paper presented at the 1958 Annual Convention of the American Psychological Association, Washington, D.C.

gressions, and that regressions and failures to progress developmentally are reflected in schizophrenia.

Sullivan[1] suggested that integrations may occur in at least five significantly different modes: the empathic, the prototaxic, the parataxic, the autistic, and the syntaxic. The direction of growth is from the former to the latter.

He did not extend this notion to cover a theory about the schizophrenias. It is the proposal of the present authors that schizophrenic persons can be described systematically at various steps along such a continuum of social maturity, with fertile implications for research and for enhanced understanding of the disease process.

## Stages of Development and Schizophrenic Integration

### *1. Empathic Stage*

*a. Problem:* The experience of anxiety.

*b. Description:* The central notion here is that anxiety has its origin in the direct discomfort felt by the infant in response to disapproval by the adult. In this early stage of life, even the crudest symbolism does not yet exist, and all experience is unconnected and discrete. Functioning is at an elementary biological level.

Emotional trauma at this stage of development tends to retard psychological growth in an extremely serious way, which is modified only by very persistent later healthy relationships.

If anxiety is persistent and severe at this empathic stage, the developmental usefulness of experience is greatly curtailed, and there may even be interference with the biological processes.

An extremely threatening aspect of anxiety in early infancy is that it cannot be evaded. The source of anxiety, usually the mother, cannot be destroyed or removed. On the contrary, the infant's usual defense, that of crying, may heighten the anxiety of the infant by heightening the anxiety of the significant adult.

At this point, another security operation may be employed by the anxiety-ridden infant, that of somnolent detachment, which serves to lessen the vulnerability of the infant by removing him from the field of interpersonal tension.

*c. Schizophrenic integration:* The adult who has been severely traumatized in the empathic stage of development tends to the most malignant species of schizophrenic behavior. The syndrome is one of a degenerative illness, usually of insidious development.

Prediction could be made that this illness will show many signs of organic dysfunction, in line with the idea that massive anxiety in the empathic period may interfere with basic biological mechanisms of living.

The prognosis here will necessarily be most unfavorable with least chance of remission. Delusional formation will tend to be profound, since the person operating with this type of integration frequently manifests infantile feelings of omnipotence in coping with the rest of the world. An enormous sum of fantasy behavior is needed to support his feelings that he is the focus of all important activity. This is the social genesis of the Kraepelinian type of schizophrenia, the so-called dementia praecox.

### *2. Prototaxic Stage*

*a. Problem:* The discrimination of discomfort in terms of direction.

*b. Description:* The prototaxic mode occurs before the young child has a self-concept as a focus of reference for experience. That is, experience is not yet differentiated in terms of formal distinctions of time or space. The child vaguely prehends earlier and later states of being without any serial connection between them. Prototaxic symbolization is that which occurs without reference to an ego, to "I" or "me."

It is in the prototaxic mode that the little child's experience of the alteration of need and satisfaction is felt. Slowly the experienced disequilibrium of need begins to be manipulated toward its alleviation by pertinent behavior, and through rudimentary symbolic processes.

There is no real movement of thought, however. Experience is discrete and unconnected. Only momentary experience is expressed by the symbolization. But it is upon these momentary stages that subsequent growth is based, so that prototaxic experience is vitally important for later experiences.

*c. Schizophrenic integration:* In view of the primitive form of symbolic conduct characteristic of this mode, and in view of the fact that no self-concept has as yet developed, the schizophrenic personality referable to this stage of development is characterized by a significant amount of magical thinking.

The grandiose schizophrenic makes claims of special power or distinction with little awareness of reality. The delusions are often supported by hallucinations and are poorly systematized. Therefore the claims are very difficult for other persons to comprehend or to share.

The Mignon delusion seems to be especially frequent in the prototaxic stage of schizophrenia because the crucial problem of this stage lies in the seeking for relief from the mothering one. That is to say that where alleviation is not to be found in the real parent, the schizophrenic person begins to cherish the belief that he is actually the kidnapped or the sole descendant of a powerful, wealthy, or high-born family. The actual parents are perceived by him as being dupes or frauds. This delusion of adoption may be elaborated upon and extended into public conduct, so that the individual is likely to assert that he was abducted as an infant by outlaws or gypsies or disgruntled domestics.

Generally there are profound disorders of thinking and communication in schizophrenics regressed to the prototaxic organization of behavior, but these are still more coherent than that of the previous level, and there is some effort on the part of the patient to define himself for others.

### 3. *Paratactic Stage*

*a. Problem:* The crystallization of a self-system.

*b. Description:* The central idea here is that the self-system becomes more evident. But what is experienced is implicitly and unreflectively assumed to be the natural way of such events. The step-by-step process of symbolic activity is not there, and inferences thus cannot be made. The state of experience is momentary and unconnected.

However, the evolving ability to symbolize enables the child to find selfhood in the behavior of others. He engages continously in a process of transfer, back and forth, between perception of others and perception of self. The self-picture mingles with the picture of significant others. In good measure, the child becomes his mother and his mother becomes himself. When father, or siblings, make their impression upon the child, they become parts of him too.

Gradually, the child is able to perceive the approval or disapproval of parents, whereas he previously only felt it. As his observation improves, his grasp of the approved and disapproved patterns of conduct becomes more refined. The child learns to focus his attention not only on the behavior which brings approval, but also on that which carries disapproval. Thus he becomes better able to avoid disapprobation by alert observation. Out of this alertness the self is first evolved. The tendency to view the self in a valuing way rather than in a devaluing way is correlated with parental approbation.

Anxiety arises from disapproval, restricting not only action, but also conscious thought. Clear thinking does not occur in matters uncongenial to the self; dissociated events are those to which the self refuses awareness and recognition.

*c. Schizophrenic integration:* In the parataxic schizophrenic state, the self-system is unable to prevent the eruption into awareness of the dissociated tendencies which could not be absorbed, even though disowned. These dissociations maintain an autonomy which is independent of the self. The result is fear and terror of inward processes which are beyond control.

An independent personification with greater power than the self is accorded to the conflict provoking tendencies. The schizophrenic operations are in this sense understood as regressive behavior attempting to protect the self. The symptomatology becomes comprehensible as efforts to regain security in the face of overwhelming threats and portents in a world become mystifying.

The world-disaster psychosis is typical of schizophrenic regressions to the parataxic mode of organization. It does not have so abruptly self-disintegrating a course as do the psychoses of the earlier stages. Frequently it is foreshadowed as a flight of panic which follows awakening during the night. The afflicted person, convinced that terrible events are transpiring, is also confused about the persons and objects in his environment.

A particularly significant combination of delusional content is one which ties together world disaster and bowel changes. Deep regression often occurs in terms of excessive preoccupation with the excreta. The patient is not only extremely untidy but is also given to coprophiliac conduct.

Generally there are nihilistic delusions to the effect that the patient is destroying everything, including himself. There is evidence of the self-system in these patients, but the defensive maneuvers are magical, bizarre, and confused. The prognosis is still unfavorable in this syndrome.

### *4. The Autistic Stage*

*a. Problem:* The development of manipulable symbols.

*b. Description:* The learning of language symbols plays a crucial part in the development of the self and the process of acculturation. In the autistic stage, the use of symbols reflects their personal and rich meaning to the individual, for the child's symbol activity is relatively unchecked by reality, and therefore is arbitrary, personal, and undisciplined.

This is necessarily so because of his limited experience with the symbol activities of others. Consensuality is lacking. The imagination of the child runs riot, since it is untested and unchecked. Yet it is in this period that the child discovers that fantasy conversations and word play enable him to respond to himself as well as to others.

The child may assume the perspectives and orientations of significant others, or he may produce the gestures of other individuals and then respond himself to these gestures. Mother, father or older sibling's roles can be played. One part is rehearsed and then another. The expectations inherent in these roles can be called out in himself. Role playing becomes a kind of safe practicing which has consequences for further social interaction, and more refined differentiation between private and public processes.

*c. Schizophrenic integration:* The person who has regressed to this stage, although his hold on reality is better than in the previous stages, is still characterized by paranoid suspiciousness, deep-lying hostilities and pathological defensiveness against his own inadequacy feelings. Furthermore, his lack of a consensually validated external group results in established habits of settling personal problems by solitary brooding.

Interpretations made by him and conclusions reached tend to become overstable since they are articulated symbolically, but are not subjected to social correction. This makes for the construction of a consistent system of delusions. All new incidents fit into this delusional organization. The schizophrenic's perceptions become highly selective.

Out of this context, the paranoid fashions an autistic pseudocommunity whose members are perceived as somehow acting against him. This, in turn, leads to conduct on the part of the patient as a reaction against the fantasied malignant acts of imagined persons, or of real persons with fantasied intentions. The patient's conviction as to the reality of this autistic community comes with abrupt clarification: a familiar declaration is that "It has all become clear to me now!"

The closure brought out by the delusionally organized pseudo-community adds considerable momentum to the further development of the system of fantasies. Once the autistic community has been formulated and crystallized, it tends to mushroom through increasingly selective perceptions of the same subjective qualities. New persons and activities are included until a position is reached where the schizophrenic views the autistic community he has erected as a serious threat to his security.

This is where he is apt to give vent to aggressive, retributory acts in the area of public behavior against his fantasied enemies. Society then meets his aggression with heavy negative sanctions like police action or institutionalization, unwittingly presenting the patient with final proof of the reality of his fears by locking him up against his will.

### 5. *The Syntaxic Mode*

*a. Problem:* The development of consensus with society.

*b. Description:* The syntaxic mode of experience is learned through the person's attempt to correct the distortions of earlier stages by checking his feelings and thoughts against those of others. As his use of the mechanism increases with age, the child gradually learns his society's patternings of relationships. He catches on to the grammatical structure of his language. Awareness increases greatly as to what to expect as a response to his verbalizations, and that these responses are agreed upon by most members of his society.

It is through this learning that the child's communications are enabled to change from autistic meanings to publicly shared ones. There comes about a concordance with others that allows fairly accurate communication by speech and gesture, and that permits the deduction of useful inference about the conduct and thinking of others.

In general, experiences which can be denoted in discussion are experiences in the syntaxic mode. In this stage of development, the person's impressions as an observer can be correlated with observed activities. New capacities for empathy and experience are formed. The more highly differentiated comprehension of what others are feeling is a process of social symbolic interaction within the child. Undistorted communications permit the achievement of open and gratifying relationships.

*c. Schizophrenic integration:* An individual at this level of functioning might become schizophrenic, but it would be a relatively circumscribed reaction. That is, the syntaxic schizophrenic is likely to be characterized by a less guarded prognosis, a relatively normal prepsychotic personality, and sudden onset with plausible environmental stresses.

Thus it is differentiated from the other modes of schizophrenia which more closely resemble each other, except that they are defined here on a maturational continuum as a way of distinguishing their varied onsets and outlooks. In short, it is suggested here that syntaxic schizophrenia occurs more or less as an appropriate reaction to accidental severe stress in normal living, such as traumatic battle experiences. The chances of repetition of breakdown in this mode tend to be minimal.

These stages have been made the basis of a life history rating procedure, in which each patient's history is rated as to the developmental level at which the life circumstances became pathological. Factors considered were such things as age at death of a parent, age of severe physical illness, age when subjected to continuing rejection, and a large number of other items, which, according to the literature, occur more frequently among schizophrenics than among normals. These life history ratings were correlated with ratings of the stage of schizophrenia. Rorschach performance scored for age level was one measure of the stage of schizophrenia. A rating of the kind of schizophrenic integration represented in the presenting psychiatric symptoms was a second measure of stage of schizophrenia. Length of hospitalization was also correlated with the life history measure. All correlations were substantial. These results lend support to the conceptualization presented above.

## Summary

To recapitulate the general approach advocated here, it is hypothesized that a fruitful empirical approach to the study of schizophrenia may be made if that dysfunction is understood as a series (or continuum) of responses that reflect the stage of development in the patient's life at which emotional support was severely deficient. Schizophrenia may be *quantitatively* described in terms of that level in life to which the schizophrenic has regressed, beyond which development was seriously distorted because of disturbing circumstances of living. The underlying psychological notion is one which proposes that the earlier in developmental history that severe stress prevails, the more damaging will be the consequences on the subsequent course of interpersonal relationships. This is not to imply that at any given point an individual's experience becomes static. What is meant is that deviations in early development may distort later growth and yield serious eccentricities in later behavior. The conceptualization is offered as an amplification and revision of the process-reactive formation.[2]

## REFERENCES

1. Sullivan, H. S., *Conceptions of Modern Psychiatry* (Washington, D.C.: William Alanson White Psychiatric Foundation, 1947).
2. Kantor, R. E., J. M. Wallner, and C. L. Winder, "Process and Reactive Schizophrenia," *Journal of Consulting Psychology,* 17 (1953), 157–62.

# 5: A Comparative-Developmental Approach to Schizophrenia

ALFRED E. GOLDMAN

There is a growing number of social and biological scientists who feel the need for a comprehensive theory of behavior—a theory of which schizophrenia in particular, or psychopathology in general, is only one facet. The theory should be broad enough to encompass data from such apparently diverse fields as anthropology, phylogenesis, human development, and states of lowered consciousness. Data from all of these areas contribute to our understanding of human behavior, and it would seem that the law of parsimony would be better served if these data could be subsumed under the same concepts and interpreted in terms of a common set of principles.

This paper attempts to outline a comparative-developmental approach to schizophrenia. It is comparative in that it relates data from the study of schizophrenia to many different fields of

Reprinted by permission of the author and publisher from *Psychological Bulletin*, 59:1 (1962), 57–69.

inquiry. It is developmental insofar as it is suggested by, and draws its basic facts from, developmental studies—the development from conception to birth, the development from childhood to adulthood, the development from the single-celled organisms to man, and from developmental studies of human cultures.

For the particular organization of the approach to schizophrenia presented here, the author accepts responsibility; the original formulation of the comprehensive comparative-developmental theory is that by Heinz Werner (1940) and his co-workers at Clark University.

Werner's comparative-developmental approach aims at viewing the total behavior of all organisms in terms of a common set of developmental principles. It is his belief that such an approach is fruitful in coordinating, within a single descriptive framework, psychological phenomena observed in phylogenesis, ontogenesis, ethnopsychology, and psychopathology. This paper confines itself to what this theoretical position has had to contribute to an understanding of schizophrenia. It attempts to indicate the comprehensiveness and heuristic value of the approach without, however, attempting to present an exhaustive review of the large body of relevant research.

Behavior proceeds through given stages in its development. A formal similarity obtains between the organization and structure of processes in young children, in organisms low on the phylogenetic scale, in human adults of technologically backward societies, and in certain states of lowered consciousness in educated normal adults of technologically advanced societies. In order for developmental theory to encompass schizophrenic processes, it requires the introduction of constructs which suggest a parallelism of various aspects of schizophrenia with developmental patterns in all of these spheres of inquiry, but especially with development in childhood. To this end developmental theorists have introduced the concept of "regression." The progression seen in the normal course of development is reversed in pathology; thus, in schizophrenia we may expect to find a regression in the direction of greater primitivization of process.

A frequently raised objection to developmental theory is that it seeks only generic similarities between various groups and tends to ignore their differences.

Exploration of developmental theory does require seeking for systematic patterns of generic similarities in cognitive performance among certain groups. Thus focused on similarities, developmental theorists have not always taken explicit account of specific differences that have appeared between groups.

The heuristic value of such an approach has already been demonstrated by the considerable number of investigations that have been provoked by or conducted under the purview of development theory. Its clinical value is suggested by its contributions to psychodiagnostic testing, in particular to the scoring and interpretation of the Rorschach technique. Genetic theory does not question that differences exist between the child and adult schizophrenic. It does hold that similarities in cognitive structure exist between young children and adult schizophrenics, both of which are exemplifications of an ideal construct; namely, developmental primitivity.

A word now about the use of the term "primitive" (Werner and Kaplan, 1956). Much of the criticism leveled at the use of this term is based on the assertion that it is moralistic in character and thus has little place in scientific endeavor. No such evaluative connotation is intended. While "primitivity" is not evaluative in this moralistic sense, it is evaluative in that it may either impede or facilitate attainment of certain goals or states. Primitivity pertains to the psychologically prior stages of development. In essence the concept of primitivity is a theoretical construct referring to a kind of cognition characterized by developmentally early processes. Processes that appear early in the development sequence—that is, early in childhood, or early in the temporal development of an idea—are more primitive than those which appear later in the sequence.

The term "regression" as used by Werner (1940) refers to the structural re-emergence of developmentally lower levels of functioning as the more advanced and more recently developed levels are disorganized. Regression in this sense differs in emphasis from the meaning given this term by psychoanalytic orthodoxy* which focuses on impulses and the methods by which these are gratified and controlled. While psychoanalysis has emphasized the *function* and *content* of psychopathology, the developmental approach considers only the *formal structure* of psychopathological processes.

By similarity in *process* between childhood and pathological primitivization reference is made to structural similarity, not to similarity in content. The regressed adult is, of course, not a child; rather, similar organizations or forms of process are identifiable in both. Our interest here is not primarily in *what* children or schizophrenics think or perceive, but rather, *how* they think or perceive. Schizophrenia thus is seen as a regression in cognitive processes; that is, it is conceived as a reversal of those patterns of thinking, perceiving, and so on, which are encountered in the normal course of development. Further, developmental theorists are not concerned with the nature of the conditions that have caused the regressed behavior or the historical antecedents of such conditions. Rather, they focus on the structural or formal consequences of these predisposing experiences.

It should be made clear that the psychoanalytic and the comparative-developmental approaches are not mutually exclusive; rather, they focus on different aspects of schizophrenia (Arieti, 1955). Each may be clinically useful and theoretically productive. Devoting attention in this paper to the structural point of view does not attribute less value or validity to the psychodynamic viewpoint. Where the psychodynamic approach is particularly helpful in therapy, the structural approach is

* Although Freud considered ego regression as well as impulse regression, many psychoanalytic practitioners are inclined to overemphasize the latter at the expense of the former.

useful in developing hypotheses, describing developmental phenomena within a consistent framework, and—most important to the clinician—it provides a gauge by which psychopathological states and modifications in those states may be assessed and understood in terms of developmental criteria (Siegel, 1953). The concept of schizophrenia which is proposed here proceeds from a basic developmental principle; wherever development takes place it initiates in a globality or lack of differentiation and becomes increasingly more differentiated, terminating in a state of integration. The development of motor coordination may serve to illustrate this developmental principle.

When stimulated, the newborn typically reacts with mass nondirected motor activity. In the normal course of maturation, this mass action becomes more focalized and better directed with respect to the stimulating agent. That is, from the total involvement of the whole body emerges a differentiated activity of certain parts of the body—arms, legs, head, and so forth. These now differentiated movements become integrated into a single smooth-flowing response in which all parts of the body may participate appropriately in achieving a goal or solving a task.

Now let us turn to the separate functions that this approach encompasses.* In each case the comparison will be made between human ontogenesis and schizophrenia.

## Emotional Behavior

Ontogenetic changes in emotional behavior proceed along at least three continua: (*a*) From overt motor expression of emotion to increasingly more internalized experience of emotion—crying (Bayley, 1932) and other motor activity decreases with age; (*b*) From globality of emotional experience to

* A comprehensive survey of developmentally oriented research in childhood may be found in Werner (1946).

greater differentiation (Bridges, 1932). At first there are only undifferentiated affective states of relative excitement or quiescence. With development there is greater specificity of emotion. For example, global negative affect becomes more differentiated into increasingly more subtle nuances, such as hate, despise, contempt, dislike, and so on. (*c*), Finally from lability of emotional experience to increased stability. In the young child there is characteristically momentary change in the nature of his emotional experiences and its expression (Jersild, 1939). What starts out as a laugh may end up in bitter tears or vice versa. Crying can be quickly changed to giggling by a well intentioned and well placed tickle.

In accordance with the regression hypothesis, in schizophrenia there is the expectation of a reversal in each of these three progressions:

1. In the acute stage of the illness, before chronicity becomes manifest in affective blunting, emotion is uncontrolled; impulse is expressed overtly without adequate intellectual intervention. Not only is the expression of affect likely to be more public, but there is an increase in the degree of motor involvement. Thus, the motoric hyperactivity of the excited schizophrenic and the motoric hypoactivity of the chronic "burnt-out" schizophrenic both exhibit the degree to which the emotional state is syncretically (Werner, 1940) fused in its expression with the motoric system. Although the affective and motoric are never wholly independent (Wolff, 1943) of each other, the immediacy, directness, and overtness of this relationship tends to increase in schizophrenia.

2. The increasing differentiation and subtlety of feelings seen in ontogenesis is reversed in schizophrenia. Clinical practice, in particular experience with the projective techniques, reflects the dedifferentiation of feelings. Aggressive and sexual components are not infrequently fused into an indistinguishable whole. Even more striking is the blatant admixture of positive and negative impulses.

3. Though perhaps not to the same degree, the emotional

experience of the acute schizophrenic is similar to that of the young child's in that it too is highly labile and unpredictable.

## Perception

The progression from globality to differentiation to integration is perhaps best seen in perception. For the neonate and very young child the visual field is not well organized or structured. Figure and ground, contours, patterns of light and shadow, movement, all merge into an undifferentiated perceptual mass, or in William James' classic terminology, "a blooming, buzzing confusion." From this globality emerge stages of increasingly differentiated perception. Here visual patterns acquire object-properties, with definitive contours and localized in three dimensional space. This development then terminates in a stage in which these differentiated aspects of the perceptual field are integrated, or synthesized, into a single meaningful percept (Werner, 1940).

This developmental sequence has been corroborated by a number of experiments, the most convincing of which have used the Rorschach blots as stimulus material (Hemmendinger, 1953). Use of this technique reveals the following changes to take place with increasing age.

Three-year-olds are whole-perceivers; they see few details and their perception is best described qualitatively in terms of their undifferentiated character. Four- and five-year-olds react less in terms of wholes and more often notice and comment on the parts. At six years another, and distinct, change occurs: an abrupt and marked increase in perceptual responses to the small and rarely noticed areas in the blots. This attraction to tiny details is interpreted as an intensification of the development of differentiation. At nine years begins the final phase of perceptual development—that of synthesis and integration. This final phase terminates in the appearance of predominantly synthesizing activity. In the integrated-whole response, the blot is perceptually articulated and then re-integrated into a well-differentiated unified whole.

Having considered perceptual development in children, we would expect, according to the regression hypothesis, a reversal of this pattern in schizophrenia. Further, we would expect that the greater the pathology the more immature the perception.

Experiments, particularly those by Friedman (1953) and Siegel (1953), reveal the following relationships in perceptual function between schizophrenics and children:

With respect to the developmentally immature response, there exists no significant difference between children and schizophrenics, and both groups differ significantly from normal adults. The same is true of the most advanced percepts. The integrated-whole response discriminates each of the three groups from each other. Thus, these findings justify the conclusion that schizophrenics, in some respects, respond perceptually in a manner similar to that of children and, in other aspects, occupy an intermediate position between normal adults and children. This may be understood in terms of the hypothetical construct of regression. In this regard regression seems evident, but it is not of such a total nature as to completely eradicate the history of the individual who has once operated on a higher developmental level.

Now, what may be said regarding the schizophrenic subtypes? There is little or no evidence on which to discriminate the perceptual functioning of the hebrephrenics and catatonics from each other, and no work has been done with simple schizophrenics. However, developmentally comparing paranoid schizophrenics with the combined hebrephrenic and catatonic group (Siegel, 1953), we find the following: While the perception of paranoid schizophrenics is typically fractionated and fragmented with emphasis on perceptual analysis, resembling the performance of children from six to ten, that of the hebrephrenic and catatonic schizophrenics is characteristic of the global, amorphous perceptual activity of three-to five-year-old children.

Comparative-developmental theory thus permits the location of catatonics, hebrephrenics, and paranoids on a developmental scale. In all aspects of cognitive functioning, in addition to perception, paranoid schizophrenics are expected to perform more like the normal adult than the catatonic or hebrephrenic schizophrenic. It does not, however, attempt to state the conditions which facilitate or inhibit the depth of regression in these diagnostic categories. At this stage in its development the theory has paid relatively little attention to motivational aspects of schizophrenia. Among clinical practitioners this conceptual vacuum has been filled by psychodynamic theories.

There are other aspects of perceptual development and regression that are instructive here:

The extreme lability that we see in primitive emotional behavior is also seen in the perceptual sphere. Those who have worked intensively with schizophrenics or with young children cannot avoid being impressed by the extreme lability of their attention. This, in both the child and in the schizophrenic, may be attributable to a kind of perceptual passivity in which competing stimuli have equal potential for evoking a perceptual response. This notion of stimuli equipotentiality may be useful in understanding the severe stimulus boundedness of the child and schizophrenic.

The child is stimulus bound in that the stimulus *must* be attended to. An infant's eyes *must* follow the hand that goes before it. His hand *must* grasp the object that is placed in it.

The schizophrenic is similarly stimulus bound. Stimuli that compete for a perceptual response cannot be adequately discriminated in terms of their relevance to a task. Thus, the schizophrenic complains of a rapidly shifting, kaleidoscopic world. A patient seen by the author complained continually that he could not attend to anything for very long because everything and anything disrupted his thoughts. Apparently irrelevant details demanded his attention: a noise outside, lights passing by at night, an apparently random thought, or a bodily sensation had equal demand on his attention as the topic being discussed or the task at hand. This extreme interpenetration of the schizophrenic's attention and thought by apparently random stimuli is a well-known phenomenon and has been well described by Cameron (1939), Kasanin (1944), and others.

## Learning

The developmental approach to learning derives from the notion that development is characterized by qualitatively different processes and modes of organization, rather than by simply quantitative variations in process. This approach is therefore in opposition to those theoretical orientations which view learning as reduceable to a single process. Developmental theory does not conceive of any one process as being paradigmatic of the whole range of human learning. A view which reduces all learning to a single process conceives of the adult as having available *more* response alternatives than the child. A genetic point of view conceives of the adult and child as utilizing *different* processes which may not be distinguishable in terms of efficiency or achievement.

Developmental theorists thus seek to understand the nature of human learning through the exploration of qualitatively distinct organizational stages. Such an exploration was undertaken in a recent study by Goldman and Denny (1963). They presented two kinds of learning tasks to children five- to fourteen-years-old. Performance in the first learning task depended on apprehending the regular pattern of the preestablished program (response to two switches in a right-right-left-left sequence). Performance in this task increased steadily with age and IQ. In the second task rewards were received according to a predetermined, random "probability" program in which one response was rewarded 25 per cent of the time and the other response was rewarded 75 per cent. Performance in this task was essentially invariant with age and IQ, with the trend somewhat favoring the younger children. Insofar as these developmental curves were strikingly different, they were interpreted as indicating that the performances on the two learning tasks reflected different processes. Insofar as the sequential, or "recursive," task required an active seeking for a general rule for its solution, it was interpreted as requiring a more advanced mode of functioning than that on the probability or "stochastic" task which permitted a more passive orientation to the task in that it did not provide for such an easily generalizable solution.

A third learning process that may represent the most primitive level for humans is classical conditioning, in which the stimulus is presented wholly at the discretion of the experimenter and the response is usually of a physiological or reflexive nature. Developmental studies of classical conditioning suggest that conditioned responses can be established very early in life and, indeed, that young children can be more easily conditioned than older children and adults (Jones, 1928, 1930 and; Kasatkin and Levikova, 1935; Mateer, 1918; Razran, 1933, 1935). The developmental primitivity of classical conditioning is further suggested by studies which indicate that susceptibility to conditioning is enhanced in states of lowered consciousness (Leuba, 1940, 1941; Scott, 1930).

Thus, at least three modes of learning are suggested which, in the order from most primitive to most advanced, are: learning by classical conditioning, stochastic learning (instrumental conditioning), and recursive learning (problem solving). The first level appears to be characteristic of the learning of very young children and of infrahuman animals. Here the learner is a kind of passive "victim" of his environment in that he does little of an active nature to learn; learning, the pairing of stimuli and response, is imposed upon him.* The second learning mode is distinguished from the first in that the learner is active or "instrumental" in the learning process, yet the learning process is essentially by rote. In this learning mode young children and adults do equally well, as do subjects of varying intelligence. The third learning mode is not only the most active in that

* A similar viewpoint was expressed by Gesell (1938).

there is a deliberate seeking for order and regularity, but there is a vigorous development and testing of solution hypotheses. This learning mode favors older and more intelligent subjects.

With growth—phylogenetic and ontogenetic—classical conditioning is less adaptive and recedes to the background until called upon—when the task situation calls for no more profound level of intellection. The other modes of learning emerge later to better serve the individual's needs.

In schizophrenia it is proposed that this development is reversed, with sequential learning and other forms of complex learning situations being affected most and classical conditioning ascending in relative importance.

Schizophrenics have been found to be more readily conditioned than normals in relatively simple situations in which the response alternatives are limited and the response reflexive. This has been demonstrated for the knee jerk (Pfaffman and Schlosberg, 1936), the psychogalvanic response (Mays, 1934; Shipley, 1934), and the eye-blink (Spence and Taylor, 1953). Schizophrenics have also been shown to exceed neurotics in eye-blink conditioning (Taylor and Spence, 1954). However, since some studies have failed to demonstrate the greater conditionability of schizophrenics over normals (Howe, 1958; Paintal, 1951), the question is raised as to what stimulus conditions enhance the establishment of the conditioned response in schizophrenics as compared to normals.

In accordance with the regression hypothesis, the increase in susceptibility to conditioning in schizophrenia should be accompanied by a decrement in performance of complex tasks. By "complex" tasks is meant tasks which permit wide response alternatives, among which are many irrelevant ones, and in which an active role of the learner is required. Schizophrenics have been found to perform poorly relative to the performance of control normals in these complex tasks (Cameron, 1939; Hanfmann, 1939; Hanfmann and Kasanin, 1942; Rapaport, 1945).

The increased conditioning performance and the decreased performance in complex tasks, in schizophrenia as compared to normals, has been interpreted by Mednick (1958) and other learning oriented theorists (e.g., Taylor and Spence, 1954) in terms of the effect of drive intensification (anxiety) on the response strength of the conditioned response. A difficulty with this type of Hullian interpretation is that it fails to take into account developmental data. The superior performance of children and infrahuman animals relative to normal adults in conditioning experiments can hardly be incorporated within such a theoretical framework unless one postulates the existence of a heightened drive state in these more primitive organisms. Genetic theory offers the parsimonious incorporation of data from all of these areas within a single theoretical structure.

When a stable stimulus-response relationship has been established the response may be elicited by other stimuli similar in some manner to the initial stimulus. This is stimulus generalization.

The genetic principle that differentiation proceeds from an initial stage of globality would suggest that in development stimulus generalization would decrease. Reiss (1946) found that young children tend to generalize readily to homophones but this tendency disappears at about 11 years of age. Mednick and Lehtinen (1957) found that amount of stimulus generalization reactivity, measured along a visual-spatial dimension of similarity, was significantly greater for younger children (7–9 years) than for older children (10–12 years).

The expectation then would be that in schizophrenia stimulus generalization would be higher than in normals of comparable intelligence. A number of studies testify that this is so (Cameron, 1938; Garmezy, 1952; Mednick, 1955).

## Thinking and Language

Thinking and language may be investigated from the vantage points of many dimensions. Three which appear to the author to be most central and inclusive are the development from idiosyncrasy to consensuality of concepts, from lability to stability of concepts, and from contextualization to autonomy of concepts.

The development from idiosyncrasy to consensuality refers to the increasingly more public and predictable thinking of which the child becomes capable as he grows older (Pollack, 1953; Werner and Kaplan, 1952). Thus, the agreement in the meaning of words among members of a given speech community increases with age. Children, in contrast to adults, use words in a private, highly individualistic manner (Hayakawa, 1954).

In psychopathological regression the development toward greater consensuality in thinking is reversed. Idiosyncratic thought then reduces the schizophrenic to virtual social isolation (Cameron, 1938; Goldman, 1960).

The second dimension is the development from lability to stability of concepts. In the young child concepts are typically labile (Pollack, 1953). The nature of the concept changes rapidly and in a seemingly capricious manner (Eng, 1931).

An example from performance on the Object Sorting Test (Rapaport, 1945) may serve to illustrate concept lability. The test consists of a number of everyday, common objects that are placed on a desk before the subject. The typical adult, when asked to place these objects into meaningful groups so that the objects within any one group belong together, will form objects into groups according to their color, or material, or perhaps their use. A subject may pick out all red objects and put them together, or all wooden objects, or all tools. Young children will frequently switch the relationship in a very labile manner (Reichard, Schneider, and Rapaport, 1944). Thus, a young child will select first a red ball and then this is placed with a red plate, the two objects having redness in common. Then a toy knife is selected because it goes on the table, too, like the red plate, and then pliers are chosen because it is metal like the knife, and then a pipe because "the workman uses the pliers and smokes a pipe."

Similar chain concepts are developed by schizophrenics in the same task situations. The response of a young schizophrenic girl in a task involving a linear schematization technique may serve as an illustration of the extreme equivocality, or lability, of the relationship between the symbol and the meaning it symbolizes (Goldman, 1960). Linear schematization requires the subject to represent a word, in this case a mood term, by drawing a line. The subject is asked to draw an "angry" line, or a line that expresses the word "misery," and so on. This subject was asked to draw a line that represented the word "healthy." She drew a series of different lines. When asked what there was in the lines she drew that suggested health she responded: "A seven upside down, lightning going up, the medusa, and this is the medical sign of health." While the patient could not clarify the way in which all of these concepts are related to health, the response invites speculation about the way each thought was related to the one that preceded it. While the experiment was in progress she was drinking 7-Up and remarked that it was "good for you." Lightning going up may represent a denial of the destructive (i.e., unhealthy) effects of lightning. The medusa may be related to "the medical sign of health" (the caduceus) by clang association, or by the snakes which are common to both.

In the extreme case, concept lability may be reflected in one word or symbol subsuming not only different concepts but opposite ones. This has been established in dreams (Jones, 1913), in archaic language (Freud, 1950), and also in schizophrenia (Goldman, 1960).

The equivocal nature of symbol meaning in childhood and in schizophrenia appears to be determined by the close bond between the symbol and some particular situation, event, or person with which it is associated. This is the third dimension—the development from contextualization to autonomy of a concept. Concepts in childhood are determined by personally relevant experience (Binet, 1916; Chodorkoff, 1952; Feifel, 1949; Hayakawa, 1954; Kasanin, 1944; Terman, 1916). A newspaper, for example, may be defined as "what the paper boy brings and you wrap the garbage with it" (Hayakawa, 1954, p. 80). With growth these concepts become increasingly independent or autonomous of these personally meaningful contexts (Werner, 1940; Werner and Kaplan, 1950, 1952).

In schizophrenia we expect the reverse of this development: concepts should become increasingly less autonomous and more contextualized. There is extensive evidence—clinical and experimental (Arieti, 1948; Baker, 1953; Cameron, 1938; Goldman, 1960; Kasanin, 1944)—that this is so. The vocabulary test performances lend further credence to the statement that in comparison to normals, schizophrenics tend to use words in terms of their concrete functions rather than in terms of abstract autonomous properties (Chodorkoff, 1952; Feifel, 1949; Harrington, 1954; Yacorzynski, 1941).

This regression may be illustrated by referring again to linear schematization. A group of schizophrenics were asked to represent the meaning of a word in a line. Then inquiry was made into the relationship between the line and the word it expressed. Typically, the line was justified in terms of some personally relevant experience. For example, the word "gentle" was represented by a patient as a haystack when she replied to the inquiry with "lying in the hay is gentle." Another patient drew two lines which she said represented the path taken by the hand of a mother "gently" caressing a child. Still a third patient represented the word "gentle" with a leaf, which "is 'gently' blowing in the breeze." Gentleness in all of these cases is represented by unique personal experiences and associations. Similarly, in the Object Sorting Test, schizophrenics are more inclined than normals to relate objects in a highly personal manner—"All of these things were in my mother's house," or, "I think they are all pretty."

Thus, three dimensions of concepts are suggested. Underlying the first, idiosyncrasy-consensuality, is the increasing stability of concepts. A concept must be stable in reference before it can be public, or consensual. Underlying, in turn, the second dimension, is the contextuality-autonomy dimension. If a concept has meaning only in terms of personal contexts, its reference will be as labile as one's personal experiences, and therefore not available for use as a vehicle for social interaction.

The second and third dimensions both reflect the developmental progress from globality to differentiation, and its dedifferentiation in psychopathological regression. To the extent that a concept is labile, or in the extreme, in that it encompasses opposite meanings, it is undifferentiated. In schizophrenia the vehicles of thinking and communication become progressively dedifferentiated in that they, the symbol and referent, are not related in a stable manner. With regard to contextualization it may be said that the more autonomous a meaning, the more it is differentiated from a particular context. Thus, in development there is progressive meaning-context differentiation, while in schizophrenia meaning and context are differentiated.

Normal subjects more frequently reflect less situational meanings and attempt to represent some essential quality of gentleness. The word "gentle" is typically symbolized by normals by a light curved line, expressing the "soft," "light" aspects of "gentle." The autonomous meaning of a word is essential in that it abstracts from each of the many situations with which it is associated (lying in hay, mother caressing child, and so on) a commonity that each shares. The essential meaning of a concept is abstracted from, but is relatively autonomous of, concrete contexts.

## Socialization

In the development of social behavior we again see the increasing differentiation out of the state of globality which terminates in integration. We have little reason to believe that in the neonate the self is distinguished from others. According to psychoanalytic theorists the mother, her breast, her voice, the warmth of her body, the sensations from within the infant's own body, are an indistinguishable whole. With development, there is an increasing awareness of the self as an entity.

The development in social integration is seen in patterns of play (Buehler, 1935; Loomis, 1931). At first, young children play in isolation with their hands, feet, or other objects. Later, children prefer to play in the presence of other children—not *with* other children, but in "parallel" play. Differentiation has taken place with this first step toward integration and will eventually lead to genuine interpersonal interaction.

This development toward social integration is also seen in the increasing complexity of the social groups, and in their increasing stability (Zaluzhni, 1930).

In schizophrenia we find similar processes, except in reverse. On the ward we can see interaction representing all of these phases. The suspicious, hostile paranoid who still seeks social interaction; the hallucinating, babbling, chronic schizophrenic who somehow still prefers to hallucinate and babble in the presence of others, although not with or in concert with others; and finally, the totally regressed isolate who withdraws into the social vacuum of a corner of the ward and devotes himself to his own bodily sensations.

## Motor Functions

One of the most striking developments to take place in the motor sphere is the increase in the implicitness of motor activity. Vicarious movements replace overt activity in reasoning, problem solving is less vocal and more silent, motion in general is less gross.

Relative to the massive debilitation in other spheres there is relatively little motor involvement in schizophrenia. It is only in the most severe regression that motor impairment is found, such as in catatonic *cerea flexibilitas,* and in the hyperactivity and restlessness that sometimes characterizes the acute stage of schizophrenia. In chronic schizophrenia, too, there is frequently evidence of incessant repetitive movements of head, trunk, or limbs.

The fact that there is little motor involvement in schizophrenia, except in severe cases, is consistent with Hughlings Jackson's principle that those functions, which are the latest to develop, are the first to be impaired in pathology. Since motor functions are among the first to develop in infancy, we would therefore expect impairment in this sphere to develop last.

There are other dimensions that have not been considered. In each of those that have been discussed, focus has been on structural similarities between young children and schizophrenic functioning. Such similarities in process are also distinguishable in primitive cultures and in states of lowered consciousness, such as dreams, drug states, and hypnogogic conditions.

A comparative-genetic approach is fruitful in our effort to understand the essential nature of schizophrenia because it seeks to expose process rather than assess achievement and it is an approach in which structure is no less important than content and function.

Although a structural point of view has been central in the systems of some theorists for some time (Arieti, 1957; Munroe, 1955; Rapaport, 1951a and b), psychoanalytic orthodoxy has not given sufficient attention to structural elements until recently. Having concerned itself in its early development predominantly with primary process, psychoanalysis is now turning increasingly more to a consideration of secondary process. Merton Gill (1959) has formalized this emphasis of the structural point of view in psychoanalysis.

This more energetic psychoanalytic consideration of ego functions and the theoretical approach that has been offered in this paper have a similar goal—the formulation of a comprehensive theory of human behavior. Such genetic approaches remind us that in our consideration of the schizophrenic, oral deprivation is a no more significant datum than is the inability to conceive of square things in terms of their squareness.

## REFERENCES

Arieti, S., "Special Logic of Schizophrenia and Other Types of Autistic Thought," *Psychiatry,* 11 (1948), 325–38.

Arieti, S., *Interpretation of Schizophrenia* (New York: Robert Brunner, 1955).
Arieti, S., "The Two Aspects of Schizophrenia," *Psychiat. Quart.*, 31 (1957), 403–16.
Baker, R. W., "The Acquisition of Verbal Concepts in Schizophrenia: A Developmental Approach to the Study of Disturbed Language Behavior" (unpublished doctoral dissertation; Worcester, Mass.: Clark University, 1953).
Bayley, Nancy, "A Study of the Crying of Infants During Mental and Physical Tests," *J. Genet. Psychol.*, 40 (1932), 306–29.
Binet, A., and T. Simon, *The Development of Intelligence in Children* (Vineland, N.J.: Training School, 1916).
Bridges, K., "Emotional Development in Early Childhood," *Child. Develpm.*, 3 (1932), 324–34.
Buehler, Charlotte, *From Birth to Maturity* (London: Routledge & Kegan Paul, 1935).
Cameron, N. S., "Reasoning, Regression and Communication in Schizophrenics," *Psychol. Monogr.*, 50 (1938), No. 1 (Whole No. 221).
Cameron, N. S., "Schizophrenic Thinking in a Problem-solving Situation," *J. Ment. Sci.*, 85 (1939), 1–24.
Chodorkoff, B., and P. Mussen, "Qualitative Aspects of the Vocabulary Responses of Normals and Schizophrenics," *J. Consult. Psychol.*, 16 (1952), 43–48.
Eng, H., *The Psychology of Children's Drawings* (London: Routledge & Kegan Paul, 1931).
Feifel, H., "Qualitative Differences in the Vocabulary Responses of Normals and Abnormals," *Genet. Psychol. Monogr.*, 39 (1949), 151–204.
Freud, S., "The Antithetical Sense of Primal Words," in E. Jones, ed., *Collected Papers* (vol. 4; London: Hogarth, 1950).
Friedman, H., "Perceptual Regression in Schizophrenia: An Hypothesis Suggested by the Use of the Rorschach Test," *J. Proj. Tech.*, 17 (1953), 171–85.
Garmezy, N., "Stimulus Differentiation by Schizophrenic and Normal Subjects under Conditions of Reward and Punishment," *J. Pers.*, 20 (1952), 253–67.
Gesell, A., "The Conditioned Reflex and the Psychiatry of Infancy," *Amer. J. Orthopsychiat.*, 8 (1938), 19–30.
Gill, M., "The Present State of Psychoanalytic Theory," *J. Abnorm. Soc. Psychol.*, 58 (1959), 1–9.
Goldman, A., "Symbolic Representation in Schizophrenia," *J. Pers.*, 28 (1960), 293–316.
Goldman, A., "Classification of Sign Phenomena," *Psychiatry*, 24 (1961), 299–306.
Goldman, A., and J. Denny, "Ontogenesis of Choice Behavior in Stochastic and Recursive Programs," *J. Genet. Psychol.*, 102 (1963), 5–18.
Goldstein, K., *The Organism* (New York: American Book, 1939).
Hanfmann, E., "Thought Disturbance in Schizophrenia as Revealed by Performance in a Picture Completion Test," *J. Abnorm. Soc. Psychol.*, 34 (1939), 249–64.

Hanfmann, E., and J. Kasanin, "Conceptual Thinking in Schizophrenia," *Nerv. Ment. Dis. Monogr.*, no. 67 (1942).

Harrington, R., and J. Ehrmann, "Complexity of Response as a Factor in the Vocabulary Performance of Schizophrenics," *J. Abnorm. Soc. Psychol.*, 49 (1954), 362.

Hayakawa, S. I., *Language in Action* (New York: Harcourt, Brace & World, 1954).

Hemmendinger, L., "Perceptual Organization and Development as Reflected in the Structure of the Rorschach Test Response," *J. Proj. Tech.*, 17 (1953), 162–70.

Howe, E. S., "GSR Conditioning in Anxiety States, Normals, and Chronic Functional Schizophrenic Subjects," *J. Abnorm. Soc. Psychol.*, 56 (1958), 183–89.

Jersild, A. T., *Child Psychology* (Englewood Cliffs, N.J.: Prentice-Hall, 1939).

Jones, E., *Papers on Psychoanalysis* (London: Bailliere, 1913).

Jones, H. E., "Conditioned Psychogalvanic Responses in Infants," *Psychol. Bull.*, 25 (1928), 183–84.

Jones, H. E. [a], "The Galvanic Skin Reflex in Infancy," *Child Develpm.*, 1 (1930), 106–10.

Jones, H. E. [b], "The Retention of Conditioned Emotional Responses in Infancy," *J. Genet. Psychol.*, 37 (1930), 485–98.

Kasanin, J. S., *The Disturbance of Conceptual Thinking in Schizophrenia* (Berkeley: University of California Press, 1944).

Kasatkin, N. I., and A. M. Levikova, "On the Development of Early Conditioned Reflexes and Differentiation of Auditory Stimuli in Infants," *J. Exp. Psychol.*, 18 (1935), 1–19.

Leuba, C., "Images as Conditioned Sensations," *J. Exp. Psychol.*, 26 (1940), 345–51.

Leuba, C., "The Use of Hypnosis for Controlling Variables in Psychological Experiments," *J. Abnorm. Soc. Psychol.*, 36 (1941), 271–74.

Loomis, A. M., "A Technique of Observing the Social Behavior of Nursery School Children," *Child. Develpm. Monogr.*, no. 5 (1931).

Mateer, F., *Child Behavior* (Boston: Badger, 1918).

Mays, L. L., "Studies of Catatonia: V. Investigation of the Perseverational Tendency," *Psychiat. Quart.*, 8 (1934), 728.

Mednick, S. A., "Distortions in the Gradient of Stimulus Generalization Related to Cortical Brain Damage and Schizophrenia," *J. Abnorm. Soc. Psychol.*, 51 (1955), 536–42.

Mednick, S. A., "A Learning Theory Approach to Research in Schizophrenia," *Psychol. Bull.*, 55 (1958), 316–27.

Mednick, S. A., and L. F. Lehtinen, "Stimulus Generalization as a Function of Age in Children," *J. Exp. Psychol.*, 53 (1957), 180–83.

Munroe, Ruth, *Schools of Psychoanalytic Thought* (New York: Dryden, 1955).

Paintal, A. S., "A Comparison of the GSR in Normals and Psychotics," *J. Exp. Psychol.*, 41 (1951), 425–28.

Pfaffman, C., and H. Schlosberg, "The Conditioned Knee Jerk in Psychotic and Normal Individuals," *J. Psychol.*, 1 (1936), 201–206.

Pollack, R. H., "A Genetic Study of Intuitive Word Meanings" (unpub-

lished doctoral dissertation; Worcester, Mass.: Clark University, 1953).
Rapaport, D. [a], "The Conceptual Model of Psychoanalysis," *J. Pers.*, 20 (1951), 56–81.
Rapaport, D. [b], *Organization and Pathology of Thought* (New York: Columbia University Press, 1951).
Rapaport, D., M. Gill, and R. Shafer, *Diagnostic Psychological Testing*, (vol. 1; Chicago: Year Book, 1945).
Razran, G., "Conditioned Responses in Children," *Arch. Psychol.*, no. 148 (1933).
Razran, G., "Conditioned Responses: An Experimental Study and a Theoretical Analysis," *Arch. Psychol.*, no. 191 (1935).
Reichard, Suzanne, Marion Schneider, and D. Rapaport, "The Development of Concept Formation in Children," *Amer. J. Orthopsychiat.*, 14 (1944), 156–61.
Reiss, B. F., "Genetic Changes in Semantic Conditioning," *J. Exp. Psychol.*, 36 (1946), 143–52.
Scott, H. D., "Hypnosis and the Conditioned Reflex," *J. Gen. Psychol.*, 4 (1930), 113–30.
Shipley, W. C., "Studies of Catatonia: VI. Further Investigation of the Perseverative Tendency," *Psychiat. Quart.*, 8 (1934), 736–44.
Siegel, E. L., "Genetic Parallels of Perceptual Structuralization in Paranoid Schizophrenia: An Analysis by Means of the Rorschach Test," *J. Proj. Tech.*, 17 (1953), 151–61.
Spence, K. W., and J. A. Taylor, "The Relation of Conditioned Response Strength to Anxiety in Normal, Neurotic, and Psychotic Subjects," *J. Exp. Psychol.*, 45 (1953), 265–77.
Taylor, J. A., and K. W. Spence, "Conditioning Level in the Behavior Disorders," *J. Abnorm. Soc. Psychol.*, 49 (1954), 497–503.
Terman, L. M., *The Measurement of Intelligence* (Boston: Houghton Mifflin, 1916).
Werner, H., *Comparative Psychology of Mental Development* (New York: Harper & Row, 1940).
Werner, H., "Genetic Experimental Psychology," in P. L. Harriman, ed., *Encyclopedia of Psychology* (New York: Philosophical Library, 1946).
Werner, H., and B. Kaplan, "The Developmental Approach to Cognition: Its Relevance to the Psychological Interpretation of Anthropological and Ethnolinguistic Data," *Amer. Anthropologist*, 58 (1956), 866–80.
Werner, H. and Edith Kaplan, "Development of Word Meaning Through Verbal Context: An Experimental Study," *J. Psychol.*, 29 (1950), 251–57.
Werner, H., and Edith Kaplan, *The Acquisition of Word Meanings: A Developmental Study* (Evanston, Illinois: Child Development, 1952).
Wolff, W., *The Expression of Personality* (New York: Harper & Row, 1943).
Yacorzynski, G. K., "An Evaluation of the Postulates Underlying the Babcock Deterioration Test," *Psychol. Rev.*, 48 (1941), 261–67.
Zaluzhni, A. S., "Collective Behavior of Children at Preschool Age," *J. Soc. Psychol.*, 1 (1930), 367–78.

# 6 Toward a Theory of Schizophrenia

GREGORY BATESON
DON D. JACKSON
JAY HALEY
JOHN WEAKLAND

This is a report on a research project that has been formulating and testing a broad, systematic view of the nature, etiology, and therapy of schizophrenia. Our research in this field has proceeded by discussion of a varied body of data and ideas, with all of us contributing according to our varied experience in anthropology, communications analysis, psycho-

Reprinted by permission of the authors and publisher from *Behavioral Science*, 1 (1956), 251–64. The following credits were cited there: "This paper derives from hypotheses first developed in a research project financed by the Rockefeller Foundation from 1952–54, administered by the Department of Sociology and Anthropology at Stanford University and directed by Gregory Bateson. Since 1954 the project has continued, financed by the Josiah Macy, Jr., Foundation. To Jay Haley is due credit for recognizing that the symptoms of schizophrenia are suggestive of an inability to discriminate the Logical Types, and this was amplified by Bateson, who added the notion that the symptoms and etiology could be formally described in terms of a double bind hypothesis. The hypothesis was communicated to D. D. Jackson and found to fit closely with his ideas of family homeostasis. Since then Dr. Jackson has worked closely with the project. The study of the formal analogies between hypnosis and schizophrenia has been the work of John H. Weakland and Jay Haley."

therapy, psychiatry, and psychoanalysis. We have now reached common agreement on the broad outlines of a communicational theory of the origin and nature of schizophrenia; this paper is a preliminary report on our continuing research.

## The Base in Communications Theory

Our approach is based on that part of communications theory which Russell has called the Theory of Logical Types.[17] The central thesis of this theory is that there is a discontinuity between a class and its members. The class cannot be a member of itself nor can one of the members *be* the class, since the term used for the class is of a *different level of abstraction*—a different Logical Type—from terms used for members. Although in formal logic there is an attempt to maintain this discontinuity between a class and its members, we argue that in the psychology of real communications this discontinuity is continually and inevitably breached,[2] and that *a priori* we must expect a pathology to occur in the human organism when certain formal patterns of the breaching occur in the communication between mother and child. We shall argue that this pathology at its extreme will have symptoms whose formal characteristics would lead the pathology to be classified as a schizophrenia.

Illustrations of how human beings handle communication involving multiple Logical Types can be derived from the following fields:

*1. The use of various communicational modes in human communications.* Examples are play, nonplay, fantasy, sacrament, metaphor, and so on. Even among the lower mammals there appears to be an exchange of signals which identify certain meaningful behavior as "play."* These signals are evidently of higher Logical Type than the messages they classify.

* A film prepared during this project, "The Nature of Play; Part I, River Otters," is available.

Among human beings this framing and labeling of messages and meaningful actions reaches considerable complexity, with the peculiarity that our vocabulary for such discrimination is still very poorly developed, and that we rely preponderantly upon nonverbal media of posture, gesture, facial expression, intonation, and the context for the communication of these highly abstract, but vitally important, labels.

2. *Humor.* This seems to be a method of exploring the implicit themes in thought or in a relationship. The method of exploration involves the use of messages which are characterized by a condensation of Logical Types or communicational modes. A discovery, for example, occurs when it suddenly becomes plain that a message was not only metaphoric but also more literal, or vice versa. That is to say, the explosive moment in humor is the moment when the labeling of the mode undergoes a dissolution and resynthesis. Commonly, the punch line compels a re-evaluation of earlier signals which ascribed to certain messages a particular mode (e.g., literalness or fantasy). This has the peculiar effect of attributing *mode* to those signals which had previously the status of that higher Logical Type which classifies the modes.

3. *The falsification of mode-identifying signals.* Among human beings mode identifiers can be falsified, and we have the artificial laugh, the manipulative simulation of friendliness, the confidence trick, kidding, and the like. Similar falsifications have been recorded among mammals.[3, 13] Among human beings we meet with a strange phenomenon—the unconscious falsification of these signals. This may occur within the self—the subject may conceal from himself his own real hostility under the guise of metaphoric play—or it may occur as an unconscious falsification of the subject's understanding of the other person's mode-identifying signals. He may mistake shyness for contempt, and so on. Indeed, most of the errors of self-reference fall under this head.

4. *Learning.* The simplest level of this phenomenon is exemplified by a situation in which a subject receives a message and acts appropriately on it: "I heard the clock strike and knew it

was time for lunch. So I went to the table." In learning experiments the analogue of this sequence of events is observed by the experimenter and commonly treated as a single message of a higher type. When the dog salivates between buzzer and meat powder, this sequence is accepted by the experimenter as a message indicating that "the dog has *learned* that buzzer means meat powder." But this is not the end of the hierarchy of types involved. The experimental subject may become more skilled in learning. He may *learn to learn*,[1, 7, 9] and it is not inconceivable that still higher orders of learning may occur in human beings.

*5. Multiple levels of learning and the Logical Typing of signals.* These are two inseparable sets of phenomena—inseparable because the ability to handle the multiple types of signals is itself a *learned* skill and therefore a function of the multiple levels of learning.

According to our hypothesis, the term "ego function" (as the term is used when a schizophrenic is described as having "weak ego function") is precisely *the process of discriminating communicational modes either within the self or between the self and others.* The schizophrenic exhibits weakness in three areas of such function: (*a*) he has difficulty in assigning the correct communicational mode to the messages he receives from other persons; (*b*) he has difficulty in assigning the correct communicational mode to those messages which he himself utters or emits nonverbally; (*c*) he has difficulty in assigning the correct communicational mode to his own thoughts, sensations, and percepts.

At this point it is appropriate to compare what was said in the previous paragraph with von Domarus'[16] approach to the systematic description of schizophrenic utterance. He suggests that the messages (and thought) of the schizophrenic are deviant in syllogistic structure. In place of structures which derive from the syllogism, Barbara, the schizophrenic, according to this theory, uses structures which identify predicates. An example of such a distorted syllogism is: "Men die. Grass dies. Men are grass." But as we see it, von Domarus' formulation is only a more precise—and therefore valuable—way of saying that schizophrenic utterance is rich in metaphor. With that generalization we agree. But metaphor is an indispensable tool of thought and expression—a characteristic of all human communication, even of that of the scientist. The conceptual models of cybernetics and the energy theories of psychoanalysis are, after all, only labeled metaphors. The peculiarity of the schizophrenic is not that he uses metaphors, but that he uses *unlabeled* metaphors. He has special difficulty in handling signals of that class whose members assign Logical Types to other signals.

If our formal summary of the symptomatology is correct and if the schizophrenia of our hypothesis is essentially a result of family interaction, it should be possible to arrive *a priori* at a formal description of these sequences of experience which would induce such a symptomatology. What is known of learning theory combines with the evident fact that human beings use *context* as a guide for mode discrimination. Therefore, we must look not for some specific traumatic experience in the infantile etiology but rather for characteristic sequential patterns. The specificity for which we search is to be at an abstract or formal level. The sequences must have this characteristic: that from them the patient will acquire the mental habits which are exemplified in schizophrenic communication. That is to say, *he must live in a universe where the sequences of events are such that his unconventional communicational habits will be in some sense appropriate*. The hypothesis which we offer is that sequences of this kind in the external experience of the patient are responsible for the inner conflicts of Logical Typing. For such unresolvable sequences of experiences, we use the term "double bind."

## *The Double Bind*

The necessary ingredients for a double bind situation, as we see it, are:

*1. Two or more persons.* Of these, we designate one, for purposes of our definition, as the "victim." We do not assume that the double bind is inflicted by the mother alone, but that it may be done either by mother alone or by some combination of mother, father, and/or siblings.

*2. Repeated experience.* We assume that the double bind is a recurrent theme in the experience of the victim. Our hypothesis does not invoke a single traumatic experience, but such repeated experience that the double bind structure comes to be an habitual expectation.

*3. A primary negative injunction.* This may have either of two forms: (*a*) "Do not do so-and-so, or I will punish you," or (*b*) "If you do not do so-and-so, I will punish you." Here we select a context of learning based on avoidance of punishment rather than a context of reward seeking. There is perhaps no formal reason for this selection. We assume that the punishment may be either the withdrawal of love or the expression of hate or anger—or most devastating—the kind of abandonment that results from the parent's expression of extreme helplessness.*

*4. A secondary injunction conflicting with the first at a more abstract level and, like the first, enforced by punishments or signals which threaten survival.* This secondary injunction is more difficult to describe than the primary for two reasons. First, the secondary injunction is commonly communicated to the child by nonverbal means. Posture, gesture, tone of voice, meaningful action, and the implications concealed in verbal comment may all be used to convey this more abstract message. Second, the secondary injunction may impinge upon any element of the primary prohibition. Verbalization of the secondary injunction may, therefore, include a wide variety of forms; for example, "Do not see this as punishment"; "Do not see me as the punishing agent"; "Do not submit to my prohibitions"; "Do not think of what you must not do"; "Do not question

* Our concept of punishment is being refined at present. It appears to us to involve perceptual experience in a way that cannot be encompassed by the notion of "trauma."

my love of which the primary prohibition is (or is not) an example"; and so on. Other examples become possible when the double bind is inflicted not by one individual but by two. For example, one parent may negate at a more abstract level the injunctions of the other.

5. *A tertiary negative injunction prohibiting the victim from escaping from the field.* In a formal sense it is perhaps unnecessary to list this injunction as a separate item since the reinforcement at the other two levels involves a threat to survival, and, if the double binds are imposed during infancy, escape is naturally impossible. However, it seems that in some cases the escape from the field is made impossible by certain devices which are not purely negative; e.g., capricious promises of love and the like.

6. Finally, the complete set of ingredients is no longer necessary when the victim has learned to perceive his universe in double bind patterns. Almost any part of a double bind sequence may then be sufficient to precipitate panic or rage. The pattern of conflicting injunctions may even be taken over by the hallucinatory voices.[14]

## *The Effect of the Double Bind*

In an Eastern religion, Zen Buddhism, the goal is to achieve Enlightenment. The Zen Master attempts to bring about enlightenment in his pupil in various ways. One of the things he does is to hold a stick over the pupil's head and say fiercely, "If you say this stick is real, I will strike you with it. If you say this stick is not real, I will strike you with it. If you don't say anything, I will strike you with it." We feel that the schizophrenic finds himself continually in the same situation as the pupil, but he achieves something like disorientation rather than enlightenment. The Zen pupil might reach up and take the stick away from the Master—who might accept this response—but the schizophrenic has no such choice since with him there is no not-caring about the relationship, and his mother's aims and awareness are not like the Master's.

We hypothesize that there will be a breakdown in any individual's ability to discriminate between Logical Types whenever a double bind situation occurs. The general characteristics of this situation are the following:

1. When the individual is involved in an intense relationship; that is, a relationship in which he feels it is vitally important that he discriminate accurately what sort of message is being communicated so that he may respond appropriately.

2. And, the individual is caught in a situation in which the other person in the relationship is expressing two orders of message and one of these denies the other.

3. And, the individual is unable to comment on the messages being expressed to correct his discrimination of what order of message to respond to; i.e., he cannot make a metacommunicative statement.

We have suggested that this is the sort of situation which occurs between the preschizophrenic and his mother, but it also occurs in normal relationships. When a person is caught in a double bind situation, he will respond defensively in a manner similar to the schizophrenic. An individual will take a metaphorical statement literally when he is in a situation where he must respond, where he is faced with contradictory messages, and when he is unable to comment on the contradictions. For example: One day an employee went home during office hours. A fellow employee called him at his home, and said lightly, "Well, how did you get *there*?" The employee replied, "By automobile." He responded literally because he was faced with a message which asked him what he was doing at home when he should have been at the office, but which denied that this question was being asked by the way it was phrased. (Since the speaker felt it wasn't really his business, he spoke metaphorically.) The relationship was intense enough so that the victim was in doubt how the information would be used, and he therefore responded literally. This is characteristic of anyone who feels "on the spot," as demonstrated by the careful literal replies of a witness on the stand in a court trial. The schizophrenic feels so terribly on the spot at all times that he habitually responds with a defensive insistence on the literal level when it is quite inappropriate; e.g., when someone is joking.

Schizophrenics also confuse the literal and metaphoric in their own utterance when they feel themselves caught in a double bind. For example, a patient may wish to criticize his therapist for being late for an appointment, but he may be unsure what sort of a message that act of being late was—particularly if the therapist has anticipated the patient's reaction and apologized for the event. The patient cannot say, "Why were you late? Is it because you don't want to see me today?" This would be an accusation, and so he shifts to a metaphorical statement. He may then say, "I knew a fellow once who missed a boat, his name was Sam and the boat almost sunk . . ." and so on. Thus he develops a metaphorical story and the therapist may or may not discover in it a comment on his being late. The convenient thing about a metaphor is that it leaves it up to the therapist (or mother) to see an accusation in the statement if he chooses, or to ignore it if he chooses. Should the therapist accept the accusation in the metaphor, then the patient can accept the statement he has made about Sam as metaphorical. If the therapist points out that this doesn't sound like a true statement about Sam, as a way of avoiding the accusation in the story, the patient can argue that there really was a man named Sam. As an answer to the double bind situation, a shift to a metaphorical statement brings safety. However, it also prevents the patient from making the accusation he wants to make. But, instead of getting over his accusation by indicating that this is a metaphor, the schizophrenic patient seems to try to get over the fact that it is a metaphor by making it more fantastic. If the therapist should ignore the accusation in the story about Sam, the schizophrenic may then tell a story about going to Mars in a rocket ship as a way of putting over his accusation. The indication that it is a metaphorical statement lies in the fantastic aspect of the metaphor, not in the signals which usually accompany metaphors to tell the listener that a metaphor is being used.

It is not only safer for the victim of a double bind to shift to a metaphorical order of message, but in an impossible situation it is better to shift and become somebody else, or shift and insist that he is somewhere else. Then the double bind cannot work on the victim because it isn't he and besides—he is in a different place. In other words, the statements which show that a patient is disoriented can be interpreted as ways of defending himself against the situation he is in. The pathology enters when the victim himself either does not know that his responses are metaphorical or cannot say so. To recognize that he was speaking metaphorically, he would need to be aware that he was defending himself and therefore was afraid of the other person. To him such an awareness would be an indictment of the other person and therefore provoke disaster.

If an individual has spent his life in the kind of double bind relationship described here, his way of relating to people after a psychotic break would have a systematic pattern. First, he would not share with normal people those signals which accompany messages to indicate what a person means. His metacommunicative system—the communications about communication—would have broken down, and he would not know what kind of message a message was. If a person said to him, "What would you like to do today?" he would be unable to judge accurately by the context or by the tone of voice or gesture whether he was being condemned for what he did yesterday, or being offered a sexual invitation, or just what was meant. Given this inability to judge accurately what a person really means and an excessive concern with what is really meant, an individual might defend himself by choosing one or more of several alternatives. He might, for example, assume that behind every statement there is a concealed meaning which is detrimental to his welfare. He would then be excessively concerned with hidden meanings and determined to demonstrate that he could not be deceived—as he had been all his life. If he chooses this alternative, he will be continually searching for meanings behind what people say and behind chance occurrences in the environment, and he will be characteristically suspicious and defiant.

He might choose another alternative and tend to accept literally everything people say to him; when their tone or gesture or context contradicted what they said, he might establish a pattern of laughing off these metacommunicative signals. He would give up trying to discriminate between levels of message and treat all messages as unimportant or something to be laughed at.

If he didn't become suspicious of metacommunicative messages or attempt to laugh them off, he might choose to try to ignore them. Then he would find it necessary to see and hear less and less of what went on around him, and do his utmost to avoid provoking a response in his environment. He would try to detach his interest from the external world and concentrate on his own internal processes and, therefore, give the appearance of being a withdrawn, perhaps mute, individual.

This is another way of saying that if an individual doesn't know what sort of message a message is, he may defend himself in ways which have been described as paranoid, hebephrenic, or catatonic. These three alternatives are not the only ones. The point is that he cannot choose the one alternative which would help him to discover what people mean; he cannot, without considerable help, discuss the messages of others. Without being able to do that, the human being is like any self-correcting system which has lost its governor; it spirals into never-ending, but always systematic, distortions.

## A Description of the Family Situation

The theoretical possibility of double bind situations stimulated us to look for such communication sequences in the schizophrenic patient and in his family situation. Toward this end we have studied the written and verbal reports of psychotherapists who have treated such patients intensively; we have studied tape recordings of psychotherapeutic interviews, both of our own patients and others; we have interviewed and taped parents of schizophrenics; we have had two mothers and one father participate in intensive psychotherapy; and we have interviewed and taped parents and patients seen jointly.

On the basis of these data we have developed a hypothesis about the family situation that ultimately leads to an individual suffering from schizophrenia. This hypothesis has not been statistically tested; it selects and emphasizes a rather simple set of interactional phenomena and does not attempt to describe comprehensively the extraordinary complexity of a family relationship.

We hypothesize that the family situation of the schizophrenic has the following general characteristics:

1. A child whose mother becomes anxious and withdraws if the child responds to her as a loving mother. That is, the child's very existence has a special meaning to the mother which arouses her anxiety and hostility when she is in danger of intimate contact with the child.

2. A mother to whom feelings of anxiety and hostility toward the child are not acceptable, and whose way of denying them is to express overt loving behavior to persuade the child to respond to her as a loving mother and to withdraw from him if he does not. "Loving behavior" does not necessarily imply "affection"; it can, for example, be set in a framework of doing the proper thing, instilling "goodness," and the like.

3. The absence of anyone in the family, such as a strong and insightful father, who can intervene in the relationship between the mother and child and support the child in the face of the contradictions involved.

Since this is a formal description, we are not specifically concerned with why the mother feels this way about the child, but we suggest that she could feel this way for various reasons. It may be that merely having a child arouses anxiety about herself and her relationships to her own family; or it may be important to her that the child is a boy or a girl, or born on the anniversary of one of her own siblings,[8] or in the same sibling position in the family that she was; or the child may be special to her for other reasons related to her own emotional problems.

Given a situation with these characteristics, we hypothesize that the mother of a schizophrenic will be simultaneously expressing at least two orders of message. (For simplicity in this presentation we shall confine ourselves to two orders.) These orders of message can be roughly characterized as (*a*) hostile or wtihdrawing behavior which is aroused whenever the child approaches her, and (*b*) simulated loving or approaching behavior which is aroused when the child responds to her hostile and withdrawing behavior, as a way of denying that she is withdrawing. Her problem is to control her anxiety by controlling the closeness and distance between herself and her child. To put this another way, if the mother begins to feel affectionate and close to her child, she begins to feel endangered and must withdraw from him; but she cannot accept this hostile act and, to deny it, must simulate affection and closeness with her child. The important point is that her loving behavior is then a comment on (since it is compensatory for) her hostile behavior and consequently it is of a different *order* of message than the hostile behavior—it is a message about a sequence of messages. Yet by its nature it denies the existence of those messages which it is about; i.e., the hostile withdrawal.

The mother uses the child's responses to affirm that her behavior is loving, and since the loving behavior is simulated, the child is placed in a position where he must not accurately interpret her communication if he is to maintain his relationship with her. In other words, he must not discriminate accurately between orders of message, in this case the difference between the expression of simulated feelings (one Logical Type) and real feelings (another Logical Type). As a result, the child must systematically distort his perception of metacommunicative signals. For example, if the mother begins to feel hostile (or affectionate) toward her child and also feels compelled to withdraw from him, she might say, "Go to bed, you're very tired and I want you to get your sleep." This overtly loving statement is intended to deny a feeling which could be verbalized as "Get out of my sight because I'm sick of you." If the child correctly discriminates her metacommunicative signals, he would have to face the fact that she both doesn't want him and is deceiving him by her loving behavior. He would be "punished" for learning to discriminate orders of messages accurately. He therefore would tend to accept the idea that he is tired rather than recognize his mother's deception. This means that he must deceive himself about his own internal state in order to support his mother in her deception. To survive with her he must falsely discriminate his own internal messages as well as falsely discriminate the messages of others.

The problem is compounded for the child because the mother is "benevolently" defining for him how he feels; she is expressing overt maternal concern over the fact that he is tired. To put it another way, the mother is controlling the child's definitions of his own messages, as well as the definition of his responses to her (e.g., by saying, "You don't really mean to say that," if he should criticize her) by insisting that she is not concerned about herself but only about him. Consequently, the easiest path for the child is to accept the mother's simulated loving behavior as real, and his desires to interpret what is going on are undermined. Yet the result is that the mother is withdrawing from him and defining this withdrawal as the way a loving relationship should be.

However, accepting mother's simulated loving behavior as real is also no solution for the child. Should he make this false discrimination, he would approach her; this move toward closeness would provoke in her feelings of fear and helplessness, and she would be compelled to withdraw. But if he then withdrew from her, she would take his withdrawal as a statement that she was not a loving mother and would either punish him for withdrawing or approach him to bring him closer. If he then approached, she would respond by putting him at a distance. *The child is punished for discriminating accurately what she is expressing, and he is punished for discriminating inaccurately—he is caught in a double bind.*

The child might try various means of escaping from this situation. He might, for example, try to lean on his father or some other member of the family. However, from our preliminary observations we think it is likely that the fathers of schizophrenics are not substantial enough to lean on. They are also in the awkward position where if they agreed with the child about the nature of the mother's deceptions, they would need to recognize the nature of their own relationships to the mother, which they could not do and remain attached to her in the *modus operandi* they have worked out.

The need of the mother to be wanted and loved also prevents the child from gaining support from some other person in the environment, a teacher for example. A mother with these characteristics would feel threatened by any other attachment of the child and would break it up and bring the child back, closer to her, with consequent anxiety when the child became dependent on her.

The only way the child can really escape from the situation is to comment on the contradictory position his mother has put him in. However, if he did so, the mother would take this as an accusation that she is unloving and both punish him and insist that his perception of the situation is distorted. By preventing the child from talking about the situation, the mother forbids him using the metacommunicative level—the level we use to correct our perception of communicative behavior. The ability to communicate about communication, to comment upon the meaningful actions of oneself and others, is essential for successful social intercourse. In any normal relationship there is a constant interchange of metacommunicative messages such as "What do you mean?" or "Why did you do that?" or "Are you kidding me?" and so on. To discriminate accurately what people are really expressing we must be able to comment directly or indirectly on that expression. This metacommunicative level the schizophrenic seems unable to use successfully.[2] Given these characteristics of the mother, it is apparent why. If she is denying one order of message, then any statement about her statements endangers her and she must forbid it. Therefore, the child grows up unskilled in his ability to communicate about communication and, as a result, unskilled in determining what people really mean and unskilled in expressing what he really means, which is essential for normal relationships.

In summary, then, we suggest that the double bind nature of the family situation of a schizophrenic results in placing the child in a position where if he responds to his mother's simulated affection her anxiety will be aroused and she will punish him (or insist, to protect herself, that *his* overtures are simulated, thus confusing him about the nature of his own messages) to defend herself from closeness with him. Thus the child is blocked from intimate and secure associations with his mother. However, if he does not make overtures of affection, she will feel that this means she is not a loving mother and her anxiety will be aroused. Therefore, she will either punish him for withdrawing or make overtures toward the child to insist that he demonstrate that he loves her. If he then responds and shows her affection, she will not only feel endangered again, but may resent the fact that she had to force him to respond. In either case in the relationship, the most important in his life and the model for all others, he is punished if he indicates love and affection and punished if he does not; and his escape routes from the situation, such as gaining support from others, are cut off. This is the basic nature of the double bind relationship between mother and child. This description has not depicted, of course, the more complicated interlocking gestalt that is the "family" of which the "mother" is one important part.[11, 12]

## ILLUSTRATIONS FROM CLINICAL DATA

An analysis of an incident occurring between a schizophrenic patient and his mother illustrates the double bind situation. A young man who had fairly well recovered from an acute schizophrenic episode was visited in the hospital by his mother. He was glad to see her and impulsively put his arm around her shoulders, whereupon she stiffened. He withdrew his arm and she asked, "Don't you love me any more?" He then blushed, and she said, "Dear, you must not be so easily embarrassed and afraid of your feelings." The patient was able to stay with her only a few minutes more and following her departure he assaulted an aide and was put in the tubs.

Obviously, this result could have been avoided if the young man had been able to say, "Mother, it is obvious that you become uncomfortable when I put my arm around you, and that you have difficulty accepting a gesture of affection from me." However, the schizophrenic patient doesn't have this possibility open to him. His intense dependency and training prevents him from commenting upon his mother's communicative behavior, though she comments on his and forces him to accept and to attempt to deal with the complicated sequence. The complications for the patient include the following:

1. The mother's reaction of not accepting her son's affectionate gesture is masterfully covered up by her condemnation of him for withdrawing, and the patient denies his perception of the situation by accepting her condemnation.

2. The statement, "Don't you love me any more," in this context seems to imply:

a. "I am lovable."

b. "You should love me and if you don't you are bad or at fault."

c. "Whereas you did love me previously you don't any longer," and thus focus is shifted from his expressing affection to his inability to be affectionate. Since the patient has also hated her, she is on good ground here, and he responds appropriately with guilt, which she then attacks.

d. "What you just expressed *was not affection,*" and in order to accept this statement the patient must deny what she and the culture have taught him about how one expresses affection. He must also question the times with her, and with others, when he thought he was experiencing affection and when they *seemed* to treat the situation as if he had. He experiences here loss-of-support phenomena and is put in doubt about the reliability of past experience.

3. The statement, "You must not be so easily embarrassed and afraid of your feelings," seems to imply:

a. "You are not like me and are different from other nice or normal people because we express our feelings."

b. "The feelings you express are all right, it's only that *you* can't accept them." However, if the stiffening on her part had indicated "These are unacceptable feelings," then the boy is told that he should not be embarrassed by unacceptable feelings. Since he has had a long training in what is and is not acceptable to both her and society, he again comes into conflict with the past. If he is unafraid of his own feelings (which mother implies is good), he should be unafraid of his affection and would then notice that it was she who was afraid, but he must not notice that because her whole approach is aimed at covering up this shortcoming in herself.

The impossible dilemma thus becomes: "If I am to keep my tie to mother I must not show her that I love her, but if I do not show her that I love her, then I will lose her."

The importance to the mother of her special method of control is strikingly illustrated by the interfamily situation of a young woman schizophrenic who greeted the therapist on their first meeting with the remark, "Mother had to get married and now I'm here." This statement meant to the therapist that:

1. The patient was the result of an illegitimate pregnancy.

2. This fact was related to her present psychosis (in her opinion).

3. "Here" referred to the psychiatrist's office and to the patient's presence on earth for which she had to be eternally indebted to her mother, especially since her mother had sinned and suffered in order to bring her into the world.

4. "Had to get married" referred to the shot-gun nature of her mother's wedding and to the mother's response to pressure that she must marry, and, reciprocally, that she resented the forced nature of the situation and blamed the patient for it.

Actually, all these suppositions subsequently proved to be factually correct and were corroborated by the mother during an abortive attempt at psychotherapy. The flavor of the mother's communications to the patient seemed essentially this: "I am lovable, loving, and satisfied with myself. You are lovable when you are like me and when you do what I say." At the same time the mother indicated to the daughter both by words and behavior: "You are physically delicate, unintelligent, and different from me ('not normal'). You need me and me alone because of these handicaps, and I will take care of you and love you." Thus the patient's life was a series of beginnings, of attempts at experience, which would result in failure and withdrawal to the maternal hearth and bosom because of the collusion between her and her mother.

It was noted in collaborative therapy that certain areas important to the mother's self-esteem were especially conflictual situations for the patient. For example, the mother needed the fiction that she was close to her family and that a deep love existed between her and her own mother. By analogy the relationship to the grandmother served as the prototype for the mother's relationship to her own daughter. On one occasion when the daughter was seven or eight years old the grandmother in a rage threw a knife which barely missed the little girl. The mother said nothing to the grandmother but hurried the little girl from the room with the words, "Grandmommy really loves you." It is significant that the grandmother took the attitude toward the patient that she was not well enough controlled, and she used to chide her daughter for being too easy on the child. The grandmother was living in the house during one of the patient's psychotic episodes, and the girl took great delight in throwing various objects at the mother and grandmother while they cowered in fear.

The mother felt herself very attractive as a girl, and she felt that her daughter resembled her rather closely, although by damning with faint praise it was obvious that she felt the daughter definitely ran second. One of the daughter's first acts during a psychotic period was to announce to her mother that she was going to cut off all her hair. She proceeded to do this while the mother pleaded with her to stop. Subsequently the mother would show a picture of *herself* as a girl and explain to people how the patient would look if she only had her beautiful hair.

The mother, apparently without awareness of the significance of what she was doing, would equate the daughter's illness with not being very bright and with some sort of organic brain difficulty. She would invariably contrast this with her own intelligence as demonstrated by her *own* scholastic record. She treated her daughter with a completely patronizing and placating manner that was insincere. For example, in the psychiatrist's presence she promised her daughter that she would not allow her to have further shock treatments, and as soon as the girl was out of the room she asked the doctor if he didn't feel she should be hospitalized and given electric shock treatments. One clue to this deceptive behavior arose during the mother's therapy. Although the daughter had had three previous hospitalizations the mother had never mentioned to the doctors that she herself had had a psychotic episode when she discovered that she was pregnant. The family whisked her away to a small sanitarium in a nearby town, and she was, according to her own statement, strapped to a bed for six weeks. Her family did not visit her during this time, and no one except her parents and her sister knew that she was hospitalized.

There were two times during therapy when the mother showed intense emotion. One was in relating her own psychotic experience; the other was on the occasion of her last visit when she accused the therapist of trying to drive her crazy by forcing her to choose between her daughter and her husband. Against medical advice, she took her daughter out of therapy.

The father was as involved in the homeostatic aspects of the intrafamily situation as the mother. For example, he stated that he had to quit his position as an important attorney in order to bring his daughter to an area where competent psychiatric help was available. Subsequently, acting on cues from the patient (e.g., she frequently referred to a character named "Nervous Ned") the therapist was able to elicit from him that he had hated his job and for years had been trying to "get out from under." However, the daughter was made to feel that the move was initiated for her.

On the basis of our examination of the clinical data, we have been impressed by a number of observations, including:

1. The helplessness, fear, exasperation, and rage which a double bind situation provokes in the patient, but which the mother may serenely and un-understandingly pass over. We have noted reactions in the father that create double bind situations, or extend and amplify those created by the mother, and we have seen the father, passive and outraged, but helpless, become ensnared in a manner similar to the patient.

2. The psychosis seems, in part, a way of dealing with double bind situations to overcome their inhibiting and controlling effect. The psychotic patient may make astute, pithy, often metaphorical remarks that reveal an insight into the forces binding him. Contrariwise, he may become rather expert in setting up double bind situations himself.

3. According to our theory, the communication situation described is essential to the mother's security and, by inference, to the family homeostasis. If this be so, then when psychotherapy of the patient helps him become less vulnerable to

mother's attempts at control, anxiety will be produced in the mother. Similarly, if the therapist interprets to the mother the dynamics of the situation she is setting up with the patient, this should produce an anxiety response in her. Our impression is that when there is a perduring contact between patient and family (especially when the patient lives at home during psychotherapy), this leads to a disturbance (often severe) in the mother and sometimes in both mother and father and other siblings.[10, 11]

## Current Position and Future Prospects

Many writers have treated schizophrenia in terms of the most extreme contrast with any other form of human thinking and behavior. While it is an isolable phenomenon, so much emphasis on the differences from the normal—rather like the fearful physical segregation of psychotics—does not help in understanding the problems. In our approach we assume that schizophrenia involves general principles which are important in all communication and therefore many informative similarities can be found in "normal" communication situations.

We have been particularly interested in various sorts of communication which involve both emotional significance and the necessity of discriminating between orders of message. Such situations include play, humor, ritual, poetry, and fiction. Play, especially among animals, we have studied at some length.[3] It is a situation which strikingly illustrates the occurrence of metamessages whose correct discrimination is vital to the cooperation of the individuals involved; for example, false discrimination could easily lead to combat. Rather closely related to play is humor, a continuing subject of our research. It involves sudden shifts in Logical Types as well as discrimination of those shifts. Ritual is a field in which unusually real or literal ascriptions of Logical Type are made and defended as vigorously as the schizophrenic defends the "reality" of his delusions. Poetry exemplifies the communicative power of metaphor—even very unusual metaphor—when labeled as such by various signs, as contrasted to the obscurity of unlabeled schizophrenic metaphor. The entire field of fictional communication, defined as the narration or depiction of a series of events with more or less of a label of actuality, is most relevant to the investigation of schizophrenia. We are not so much concerned with the content interpretation of fiction—although analysis of oral and destructive themes is illuminating to the student of schizophrenia—as with the formal problems involved in simultaneous existence of multiple levels of message in the fictional presentation of "reality." The drama is especially interesting in this respect, with both performers and spectators responding to messages about both the actual and the theatrical reality.

We are giving extensive attention to hypnosis. A great array of phenomena that occurs as schizophrenic symptoms—hallucinations, delusions, alterations of personality, amnesias, and so on—can be produced temporarily in normal subjects with hypnosis. These need not be directly suggested as specific phenomena, but can be the "spontaneous" result of an arranged communication sequence. For example, Erickson[4] will produce a hallucination by first inducing catalepsy in a subject's hand and then saying, "There is no conceivable way in which your hand can move, yet when I give the signal, it must move." That is, he tells the subject his hand will remain in place, yet it will move, and in no way the subject can consciously conceive. When Erickson gives the signal, the subject hallucinates the hand moved, or hallucinates himself in a different place and therefore that the hand was moved. This use of hallucination to resolve a problem posed by contradictory commands which cannot be discussed seems to us to illustrate the solution of a double bind situation via a shift in Logical Types. Hypnotic responses to direct suggestions or statements also commonly involve shifts in type, as in accepting the words, "Here's a glass of water," or "You feel tired" as external or internal reality, or in literal response to metaphorical statements, much like schizophrenics. We hope that further study of hypnotic induction, phenomena, and waking, will—in this controllable situation—help sharpen our view of the essential communicational sequences which produce phenomena like those of schizophrenia.

Another Erickson experiment[12] seems to isolate a double bind communicational sequence without the specific use of hypnosis. Erickson arranged a seminar so as to have a young chain smoker sit next to him and to be without cigarettes; other participants were briefed on what to do. All was ordered so that Erickson repeatedly turned to offer the young man a cigarette but was always interrupted by a question from someone so that he turned away "inadvertently" withdrawing the cigarettes from the young man's reach. Later another participant asked this young man if he had received the cigarette from Dr. Erickson. He replied, "What cigarette?" This showed clearly that he had forgotten the whole sequence, and even refused a cigarette offered by another member, saying that he was too interested in the seminar discussion to smoke. This young man seems to us to be in an experimental situation paralleling the schizophrenic's double bind situation with mother: an important relationship, contradictory messages (here of giving and taking away), and blocked—because there was a seminar going on, and anyway it was all "inadvertent." And note the similar outcome: amnesia for the double bind sequence and reversal from "He doesn't give" to "I don't want."

Although we have been led into these collateral areas, our main field of observation has been schizophrenia itself. All of us have worked directly with schizophrenic patients and much of this case material has been recorded on tape for detailed study. In addition, we are recording interviews held jointly with patients and their families, and we are taking sound motion pictures of mothers and disturbed, presumably preschizophrenic, children. Our hope is that these operations will provide a clearly evident record of the continuing, repetitive double binding which we hypothesize goes on steadily from infantile beginnings in the family situation of individuals who become schizophrenic. This basic family situation, and the overtly communicational characteristics of schizophrenia, have been the major focus of this paper. However, we expect our concepts and some of these data will also be useful in future work on other problems of schizophrenia, such as the variety of other symptoms, the character of the "adjusted state" before schizophrenia becomes manifest, and the nature and circumstances of the psychotic break.

## Therapeutic Implications of This Hypothesis

Psychotherapy itself is a context of multi-level communication, with exploration of the ambiguous lines between the literal and metaphoric, or reality and fantasy, and indeed, various forms of play, drama, and hypnosis have been used extensively in therapy. We have been interested in therapy and, in addition to our own data, we have been collecting and examining recordings, verbatim transcripts, and personal accounts of therapy from other therapists. In this we prefer exact records since we believe that how a schizophrenic talks depends greatly, though often subtly, on how another person talks to him; it is most difficult to estimate what was really occurring in a therapeutic interview if one has only a description of it, especially if the description is already in theoretical terms.

Except for a few general remarks and some speculation, however, we are not yet prepared to comment on the relation of the double bind to psychotherapy. At present we can only note:

1. Double bind situations are created by and within the psychotherapeutic setting and the hospital milieu. From the point of view of this hypothesis we wonder about the effect of medical "benevolence" on the schizophrenic patient. Since hospitals exist for the benefit of personnel as well as—as much as—more than—for the patient's benefit, there will be contra-

dictions at times in sequences where actions are taken "benevolently" for the patient when actually they are intended to keep the staff more comfortable. We would assume that whenever the system is organized for hospital purposes and it is announced to the patient that the actions are for *his* benefit, then the schizophrenogenic situation is being perpetuated. This kind of deception will provoke the patient to respond to it as a double bind situation, and his response will be "schizophrenic" in the sense that it will be indirect and the patient will be unable to comment on the fact that he feels that he is being deceived. One vignette, fortunately amusing, illustrates such a response. On a ward with a dedicated and "benevolent" physician in charge there was a sign on the physician's door which said "Doctor's Office. Please Knock." The doctor was driven to distraction and finally capitulation by the obedient patient who carefully knocked every time he passed the door.

2. The undertaking of the double bind and its communicative aspects may lead to innovations in therapeutic technique. Just what these innovations may be is difficult to say, but on the basis of our investigation we are assuming that double bind situations occur consistently in psychotherapy. At times these are inadvertent in the sense that the therapist is imposing a double bind situation similar to that in the patient's history, or the patient is imposing a double bind situation on the therapist. At other times therapists seem to impose double binds, either deliberately or intuitively, which force the patient to respond differently than he has in the past.

An incident from the experience of a gifted psychotherapist illustrates the intuitive understanding of a double bind communicational sequence. Dr. Frieda Fromm-Reichmann[5] was treating a young woman who from the age of seven had built a highly complex religion of her own, replete with powerful Gods. She was very schizophrenic and quite hesitant about entering into a therapeutic situation. At the beginning of the treatment she said, "God R says I shouldn't talk with you." Dr. Fromm-Reichmann replied, "Look, let's get something into the record. To me God R doesn't exist, and that whole world of yours doesn't exist. To you it does, and far be it from me to think that I can take that away from you, I have no idea what it means. So I'm willing to talk with you in terms of that world, if only you know I do it so that we have an understanding that it doesn't exist for me. Now go to God R and tell him that we have to talk and he should give you permission. Also you must tell him that I am a doctor and that you have lived with him in his kingdom now from seven to sixteen—that's nine years—and he hasn't helped you. So now he must permit me to try and see whether you and I can do that job. Tell him that I am a doctor and this is what I want to try."

The therapist has her patient in a "therapeutic double bind." If the patient is rendered doubtful about her belief in her god then she is agreeing with Dr. Fromm-Reichmann, and is admitting her attachment to therapy. If she insists that God R is real, then she must tell him that Dr. Fromm-Reichmann is "more powerful" than he—again admitting her involvement with the therapist.

The difference between the therapeutic bind and the original double bind situation is, in part, the fact that the therapist is not involved in a life and death struggle himself. He can therefore set up relatively benevolent binds and gradually aid the patient in his emancipation from them. Many of the uniquely appropriate therapeutic gambits arranged by therapists seem to be intuitive. We share the goal of most psychotherapists who strive toward the day when such strokes of genius will be well enough understood to be systematic and commonplace.

## REFERENCES

1. Bateson, G., "Social Planning and the Concept of 'Deutero-learning,'" *Conference on Science, Philosophy and Religion, Second Symposium* (New York: Harper & Row, 1941).

2. Bateson, G., "A Theory of Play and Fantasy," *Psychiatric Research Reports*, 2 (1955), 39–51.
3. Carpenter, C. R., "A Field Study of the Behavior and Social Relations of Howling Monkeys," *Comp. Psychol. Monogr.*, 10 (1934), 1–168.
4. Erickson, M. H., in personal communication, 1955.
5. Fromm-Reichmann, F., in personal communication, 1956.
6. Haley, J., "Paradoxes in Play, Fantasy and Psychotherapy," *Psychiatric Research Reports,* 2 (1955), 52–58.
7. Harlow, H. F., "The Formation of Learning Sets," *Psychol. Rev.*, 56 (1949), 51–65.
8. Hilgard, J. R., "Anniversary Reactions in Parents Precipitated by Children," *Psychiatry,* 16 (1953), 73–80.
9. Hull, C. L., *et al.*, *Mathematico-Deductive Theory of Rote Learning* (New Haven: Yale University Press, 1940).
10. Jackson, D. D., "An Episode of Sleepwalking," *J. Amer. Psychoanal. Assn.*, 2 (1954), 503–508.
11. Jackson, D. D., "Some Factors Influencing the Oedipus Complex," *Psychoanal. Quart.*, 23 (1954), 566–81.
12. Jackson, D. D., "The Question of Family Homeostasis" (paper presented at the American Psychiatric Association Meeting, St. Louis, May 7, 1954).
13. Lorenz, K. Z., *King Solomon's Ring* (New York: T. Y. Crowell, 1952).
14. Perceval, J., *A Narrative of the Treatment Experienced by a Gentleman during a State of Mental Derangement, Designed to Explain the Causes and Nature of Insanity*, etc. (London: Effingham Wilson, 1836 and 1840).
15. Ruesch, J., and G. Bateson, *Communication: The Social Matrix of Psychiatry* (New York: W. W. Norton, 1951).
16. von Domarus, E., "The Specific Laws of Logic in Schizophrenia," in J. S. Kasanin, ed., *Language and Thought in Schizophrenia* (Berkeley: University of California Press, 1944).
17. Whitehead, A. N., and B. Russell, *Principia Mathematica* (Cambridge University Press, 1910).

# 7 : Cultural Isolation and the Schizophrenic Personality

ROBERT E. L. FARIS

A great forward stride in the understanding of human behavior was made when we began to study mental disorders from the medical point of view. There were many remarkable successes. When the physician found that he could explain some forms of insanity by locating injuries, glandular abnormalities, or germs, the result was the substitution of the more merciful and hopeful medical treatment for the exorcisms or punishments of the priests. It would be difficult to overstate the importance of the medical research on abnormal behavior. And yet it is an interesting fact that the one form of mental disorder that is most common in the hospitals of this country is still largely a mystery to the physician. Although a large number of studies have been made, this disorder, schizophrenia, seems to keep its secrets from those who use the medical ap-

Reprinted with the permission of the author and publisher from *American Journal of Sociology,* 40 (1934), 155–64.

proach. It is possible that the causes of schizophrenia are not to be sought primarily in the physiological mechanism but in the nature of the social relations of the person. If that is the case, the solution of the problem can never be reached through intensive study of the physiology and pathology of the individual alone. In this paper are presented the results of a study of schizophrenia from the sociological approach. It may be that through this type of study a number of the unsolved problems in the field of insanity will be cleared up.

In the books and articles that deal with this disorder, schizophrenia is not clearly defined. There is so much confusion in the literature that one may well doubt that the different authors are writing about the same phenomenon. Yet, it is possible to get something which is common to most of the accounts, and to describe the type of behavior which is the object of this inquiry. It must be borne in mind that schizophrenic patients have at least as much individuality as normal persons; and any statement about them must refer to essential characteristics of the mental disorder or the problem will be even more complicated.

The schizophrenic shows a marked divergence from the normal person in the way he thinks, acts, and feels. The actions are markedly eccentric, the habits of thought appear to lack logic, or to have a special logic of their own. The emotions of the schizophrenic frequently appear to be entirely inappropriate to the situation. Traditionally these forms of abnormal behavior have been described by such words as "hallucinations," "delusions," "impulsiveness," "inappropriate emotional states," and so on, but all show some marked deviation from conventional or normal ways of acting, or thinking, or feeling. Another characteristic said to be common to all or nearly all schizophrenics (with the exception of the catatonic type) is the seclusive, or the "shut-in," personality. The schizophrenic appears to prefer to be alone, to shun companionship, to lack sociability. Both of these characteristics, the eccentric behavior and the seclusiveness, are so striking as to make it appear that there must be something lacking in the constitutional makeup of the individual. Much of the study of this condition has been a search for the defect or the missing part, the discovery of which seemed necessary to explain the disorder.

The study of the causes of schizophrenia has been made from various points of view. Causes have been sought in heredity, germ diseases, glandular disorders, blood chemistry, brain defects, and other constitutional traits. It is safe to state that no conclusive findings have resulted from any of these approaches. In each case the findings have been enough to encourage the student to feel that further investigation might be desirable, but the net result of these studies is not impressive.

The hypothesis offered in this paper differs from the others in that the cause of schizophrenia is sought in the social experiences of the individual. It may be that the explanation lies in the nature of these experiences, and the type of social relations or the lack of social relations. Briefly, the hypothesis is that the cause of schizophrenia is isolation of the person. Any form of isolation that cuts the person off from intimate social relations for an extended period of time may possibly lead to this form of mental disorder. The eccentric behavior is the result of the seclusiveness of the person, and the seclusiveness is the result of the long period of isolation. The isolation may not be voluntary, and indeed seems to be rarely, if ever, of the individual's own choice, but, rather, due to circumstances beyond his control. Typically, the isolated person makes a struggle to establish intimate social relations, and feels lonely when he fails. In the beginning of the process the "seclusiveness" or "shut-in" trait is not the cause, but the result, of the isolation. The other eccentricities follow from this exclusiveness.

Before presenting the evidence supporting this hypothesis it is appropriate to examine the process by which the seclusiveness causes the extreme forms of eccentric behavior, thought, and feeling. Perhaps the most common explanation at the present time is that for the schizophrenia patient the world of "reality" is too unpleasant and painful to face. The "disease" is a protective device into which the patient can flee. Schizophrenia is frequently characterized as a "flight from reality."

The unconventional and eccentric behavior may be thought of as a form of "indifference to communication." Our actions are conventional because of our participation in the primary-group life of our communities. What order we can detect in human minds is principally the result of the necessity to communicate with those friends and neighbors. As long as a person wishes to appear sensible, and fears gossip, ridicule, and the sneers of his fellows, he must accept the roles defined for him by his community, and must think and feel in harmony with the attitudes and sentiments of his neighbors. To most normal people this conformity is second nature. It is so much a part of their habits that they do not sense the social control that has molded them and continues to enforce conformity to the patterns. When anything interferes with these forms of social control, there is nothing to keep the actions of the person conventional. When there is no longer any necessity or desire to communicate with others, or to appear reasonable to them, there is nothing to preserve the order in the mental life of the person. "Indifference to communication" allows "mental disorder," merely because only the necessity to communicate with, and appear sensible to, other persons preserves the "order" of a normal mind. It should be pointed out here that intensive study of schizophrenic patients indicates that "mental disorder" is not always an accurate description of the condition. The minds appear disordered, but there may be an organization there. The appearance of disorder is due to the fact that the patient makes no attempt to communicate that organization, and the normal mind is unable to discover it from casual external observation. Perhaps "mental eccentricity" or "mental unconventionality" would be a more appropriate concept than "mental disorder."

The eccentricity of the patient, then, might be considered as one result of his freedom from the informal social control of the community. The seclusiveness of his personality is enough to break down this control, for the unwillingness to communicate and appear sensible, or the feeling that it is impossible, will make a person unresponsive to this control.

"Illogical thought" is the result of the same condition of isolation. This term is probably not an accurate description either, in that it implies that the patient has lost the ability to use logic. The real truth is that he is indifferent to logic because he has no need for it. Most normal people have dreams and daydreams and indulge in thinking which has little or no logic. What logic they do use is made necessary by the desire to be understood. When there is no desire to be understood, or no hope of being understood, there is no need for the use of logic. Again, it must be remembered that this does not imply that there is no order in the mental life of the schizophrenic. It might be said that the patient has a special logic of his own, but that it is difficult to discover.

Similarly the false beliefs, or delusions, of schizophrenia are better understood if considered as mere unconventional behavior. What persons do not have false beliefs? It is not the fact that his beliefs are false that makes the schizophrenic conspicuous; it is the fact that he is alone in his belief. If three hundred people at a camp meeting see and hear the devil, they are not called schizophrenic. But if a person is certain that he is being pursued by a devil that no one else can see, he is said to have a delusion. Further intensive inquiry into these delusions usually shows that, although the person is in error, he is usually not without some basis for his belief. If he feels that he is being persecuted, it is frequently true that he suffers repeated failures, but his view of his situation is likely to be distorted. If he feels electricity going through his body, it may be true that he feels something but is mistaken in thinking that it is electricity. If he hears voices calling him names, he is sometimes able to distinguish them from voices calling out loud; they are often, in fact, a sort of "silent whisper." His interpretation may be false, but the basis for the abnormality is not its falseness but its unconventionality.

The so-called "inappropriate emotional states" which are also common among the schizophrenics are also merely forms of unconventionality. In the mind of the patient events have a significance different from the conventional. The emotions are inappropriate to the surroundings as viewed by his observers, but not to his surroundings as interpreted in his own mental organization. This and all the other forms of eccentricity characteristic of the schizophrenic may be merely due to the fact that his seclusiveness has cut him off from the social control which enforces conformity with the patterns of thought and action and feeling which are conventional and therefore normal.

The seclusiveness or the "shut-in" trait is frequently considered to be due to some innate personality defect or to some constitutional defect. It can be shown, however, that many schizophrenics were at one time sociable and fond of companionship. The seclusiveness is frequently the last stage of a process that began with exclusion or isolation which was not the choice of the patient. In the early stages the patient disliked the isolation and fought against it. He felt lonely and sought to re-establish intimate social contacts. Only after an extended period of this enforced isolation did the patient give up the struggle and become adjusted to the condition. It is typical that at this time he began to prefer his solitude and became genuinely seclusive.

Some good examples of this process can be found in the cases of prisoners who have been held in solitary confinement for long periods of time. From the data available it appears that the results of this experience are strikingly similar. Maurice Small writes that the long-term prisoners show little joy when their sentences expire. Frequently they desire to return to their cells.[1] Viera Figner tells of her long imprisonment during which she finally lost her desire to have visitors, even her mother. She no longer wanted to talk; she had to summon all her strength of will to speak when she received the infrequent visits from her mother.[2] Hobhouse and Brockway state that the effect of the separation of prisoners and the silence rule was to bring about a high rate of insanity.[3] Ives reports the same results at the Pentonville prison when the solitude treatment was tried about the middle of the last century.[4] The eccentricities the prisoners developed were of various sorts, but they were nearly all described as "thoughtful, subdued, and languid."

Sheepherders and other isolated persons are said to develop similar traits after a long period of enforced solitude. Gettys states that the typical herder in Texas avoids companionship and does not like to converse with others, and is generally cross and irritable.[5]

The schizophrenics, however, are for the most part neither prisoners nor sheepherders. It is not necessary that there be spatial separation. Cultural isolation—that is, lack of intimate social contacts—may also cause the same type of seclusiveness. The interference with social contacts may be due to various factors, but similar effects are widely observed wherever the isolation is continued for a long time. Krueger and Reckless present a case of a boy who was told that he had an ugly mouth.[6] He hadn't noticed it before, but he looked in a mirror, decided it must be true, and became sensitive, touchy, unsure of himself. When anybody looked at him, he wanted to run. He didn't believe anybody could really like him. It is typically this sort of experience which defines the role of a person—a casual remark, an adjustment in the inner life, events likely to pass unnoticed even by his most intimate associates. It is not remarkable that these associates are able to see no explanation for the personality change in the situation and experience of their friend, and are disposed to believe that there must have been some constitutional breakdown.

Kimball Young presents a case of a boy who became sensitive about his appearance because of acne on his face.[7] He became despondent, afraid of ridicule, convinced that he was regarded as disfigured and inferior. He avoided making friends and distrusted those who approached him, for he felt that it must be impossible for anyone to like him for himself and that they must have some ulterior motives. In high school he gained the reputation for being snobbish and aloof, although he always longed to be intimate with his schoolmates. Ordinarily, however, such cases as these do not become serious enough to develop into real "shut-in" types. They make friends in time, perhaps much more slowly than most persons, but ordinarily will be able to gain sufficient social contacts. But if they happen to be in a situation in which it is much more difficult to establish social contacts, even for a very sociable person, this type may never succeed. In the mobile rooming-house districts and hobo areas in the large cities, and in the slums, it might be so difficult that a person who once develops a little sensitivity, or becomes uncertain of his status, may never re-establish intimate social contacts, and thus be as isolated as the prisoner in his solitary confinement cell, and with a similar result.

Some cases gathered from the records of a hospital in Chicago illustrate the relationship between the community life and the isolation of the person. A Jewish boy was brought up in a region which was invaded by the Negro population. His mother operated a store in which they also lived, so they were not able to move. Although he went to school, the boy did not care to play with the colored boys, and so had no friends or playmates. He became interested in reading, music, and daydreaming. All his experiences with people conspired to shut him further within himself. Eventually he was brought to the hospital, where he was diagnosed as a schizophrenic.

A young woman immigrant from Czechoslovakia worked as a waitress and lived in a slum district in Chicago. She married a man from her own country and soon grew fat and bore several children. She did not learn English and consequently could not talk with her neighbors, and did not like to visit with the friends of her husband because they teased her for being fat. She became increasingly seclusive and eccentric, until finally it became necessary to send her to the hospital.

A chubby, pink-cheeked boy with reddish hair worn in long curls was teased as a "sissy" on the first day of school. He went home crying. He lived in a slum neighborhood, and the boys were of the type that do not tolerate effeminacy. The more he was teased the more he withdrew from them, and was as a consequence further excluded by them. When he left school and found a position with a large firm, he sought to establish friendships with the young men of his own age who had not known him in school. But he did not know how to approach them, and clumsily offered to treat them to refreshments and entertainment. He came to be regarded as "queer" and was avoided. He tried even more desperately by spending larger sums of money. Embezzlements for this purpose led to his arrest; and because he could not explain his actions, he was taken to the hospital and diagnosed as a case of schizophrenia.

These are typical cases. The sensitivity, according to this hypothesis, is the result of a particular experience or of several experiences, usually so trivial that they pass unnoticed by others. The rest of the process is a vicious circle—an interaction between a person already unsure of himself, and a social situation in which it is unusually difficult to establish friendships. It is in this sort of community that most cases of schizophrenia develop. In Chicago, the high rates for this disorder are sharply concentrated in the hobo, rooming house, and most deteriorated slum areas.[8] The heterogeneity and the mobility of the population greatly increase the cultural isolation of the person, and in this manner produce breeding grounds for schizophrenia. The process appears to operate about equally on all races and nationalities that inhabit these areas. The Negroes inhabit a district which extends from the center of the city all the way to the outlying residential areas. In the central part, which is a slum district, the schizophrenia rate is extremely high. In each successive district farther from the center the rate is lower, and in the residential district it is as low as the rate for the white races in the surrounding residential districts.

If it is true that schizophrenia only develops where the social situation allows it, a check on this hypothesis can be made by examining cultures in which isolation of this sort would be impossible. Some of the preliterate societies fit this description. In those societies which have little or no contact with other peoples, in which the membership is homogeneous and the social life very intimate, there could hardly exist eccentric individuals. Ellsworth Faris observed that among some of the Bantu peoples in central Africa there is no disobedience, no violation of the folkways and mores, no punishment, and the children do not even make mistakes in grammar. The informal social control is so strong that a withered old woman can give orders to the strong young men of the village. In such a situation the "shut-in" personality type would not be expected to be found. On his expedition to this country in 1932-33 Ellsworth Faris made a careful inquiry on this point. The result was that he failed to find anyone who had ever heard of such a personality type.[9] Data on other primitive communities is scarce, but there is some evidence that among the Papuans of British New Guinea there are no disorders of the schizoid type.[10] The natives of the Brazilian interior are said to have disorders of the extraverted type, but rarely of the schizoid type.[11] It is interesting that in her study of the Samoans Margaret Mead observed a few cases of assorted disorders, including one which resembled catatonic dementia praecox, but none of the "shut-in" type.[12] It should be mentioned, however, that schizoid types may be found among some primitive peoples, where the social situation is of the sort that would favor isolation.

Some evidence from still another source should be included here. If isolation is the cause of schizophrenia, the re-establishment of intimate social contacts might be expected to improve the patient. Such attempts have been made by H. S. Sullivan and also by L. C. Marsh. Sullivan encouraged comradeships between his attendants and their patients and discovered that as the genuine friendships sprung up the alleged apathy of the schizophrenic faded and the recovery rate became high.[13] Marsh used a slightly different method. He arranged a series of meetings of the patients, at which certain activities and programs were devised for the purpose of obtaining their interest and building up a social life among them. He also reports an encouraging degree of success.[14]

It cannot be said that any of the foregoing proof is conclusive. On each of the points mentioned in the discussion more data are needed. The case histories in hospital records are seldom adequate for this purpose. Good descriptions of the behavior of prisoners in solitary confinement are rare. The study of the distribution of mental disorders in Chicago needs to be repeated in other cities. More data on preliterate societies are needed. Experiments with methods of treatment might also furnish valuable evidence. Yet, the fact that all these data point to the same conclusion is, it seems, sufficiently impressive to make it worthwhile to continue investigations in the hope of resolving one of our most difficult problems.

## REFERENCES

1. Maurice Small, "On Some Psychical Relations of Society and Solitude," *Pedagogical Seminary*, 7:2 (April 1900), 42.
2. Viera N. Figner, *Memoirs of a Revolutionist* (New York: 1927), p. 29.
3. S. Hobhouse and A. F. Brockway, *English Prisons Today* (London: 1922), p. 583.
4. George Ives, *History of Penal Methods* (New York: 1914), pp. 186–87.
5. C. A. Dawson and W. E. Gettys, *An Introduction to Sociology* (New York: 1929), p. 605.
6. E. T. Krueger and W. C. Reckless, *Social Psychology* (New York: 1931), p. 340.
7. Kimball Young, *Source Book for Social Psychology* (New York: A. Knopf, 1927), pp. 360–61.
8. A number of checks on this point have been made. A full discussion is made in a manuscript by H. W. Dunham and the writer. Although there is always the possibility of revision, it seems that the interpretation of the concentration of cases is that it is because of the nature of the social situation in these areas that schizophrenia develops. One of the most interesting checks is the distribution of the catatonic schizophrenia cases. The catatonic type is not characteristically "shut-in" or seclusive. If the hypothesis is correct, there

would be no reason to expect that the catatonic rates would be concentrated in the same areas as the rest of the schizophrenic cases. As a matter of fact, they are not, and instead of being concentrated in the central slum and rooming-house districts, they are concentrated in those areas which are frontiers between the immigrant settlements and the residential districts of the native born. There is some evidence that these catatonic cases represent the American-born children of foreign parents, and are in transition from the Old World culture to the American culture.

9. Ellsworth Faris, "Culture and Personality among the Forest Bantu," *Proceedings of the American Sociological Society*, 28 (1934), 10.
10. C. G. Seligman, "Temperament, Conflict and Psychosis in a Stone-age Population," *British Journal of Medical Psychology*, 9 (1929), 187–202.
11. Lopes, C., "Ethnographische Betrachtungen uber Schizophrenie," *Zeitschrift f. d. Ges. Neur. und Psychiat.*, 142 (1932), 706–11.
12. Mead, Margaret, *Coming of Age in Samoa* (New York: William Morrow, 1928), pp. 278–81.
13. Sullivan, H. S., "Schizophrenic Individuals as a Source of Data for Comparative Investigation of Personality," *Second Colloquium on Personality Investigation* (delivered in New York: 1930).
14. Marsh, L. C., "Group Treatment of the Psychoses by the Psychological Equivalent of the Revival," *Mental Hygiene*, 15 (April 1931), 328–49.

# *Author Index*

# Subject Index